Social Work Ethics
on the Line

Social Work Ethics on the Line

Charles S. Levy, DSW

This edition published 2012 by Routledge

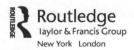

Routledge
Taylor & Francis Group
711 Third Avenue
New York, NY 10017

Routledge
Taylor & Francis Group
2 Park Square, Milton Park
Abingdon, Oxon OX14 4RN

Social Work Ethics on the Line has also been published as Administration in Social Work.

© 1993 by The Haworth Press, Inc. All rights reserved.

First published by
The Haworth Press, Inc., 10 Alice Street, Binghamton, NY 13904-1580

This edition published 2012 by Routledge

Routledge
Taylor & Francis Group
711 Third Avenue
New York, NY 10017

Routledge
Taylor & Francis Group
2 Park Square, Milton Park
Abingdon, Oxon OX14 4RN

Library of Congress Cataloging-in-Publication Data

Levy, Charles S., 1919-
    Social work ethics on the line / Charles S. Levy.
        p.   cm.
    Includes bibliographical references and index.
    ISBN 1-56024-283-3
    1. Social workers – Professional ethics – United States. 2. Social service – Moral and ethical aspects. I. Title.
HN10.5.L47 1992
174′.936232 – dc20
                                                                                    92-3349
                                                                                    CIP

CONTENTS

ABOUT THE AUTHOR

Charles S. Levy, DSW, is Professor Emeritus of Social Work at Yeshiva University. He has had many years of experience in social work practice, supervision, administration, and education. This experience has inspired and reinforced his interest in professional ethics. Dr. Levy chaired the Task Force on Ethics that produced the version of the Code of Ethics of the National Association of Social Workers adopted in 1979 and still in force today. He also chaired the NASW Ethics Advisory Panel. Dr. Levy is a member of the National Association of Social Workers and the Council on Social Work Education.

Foreword

How seasonable that Charles S. Levy should free the conceptions of ethical behavior for social workers from the morass of unethical influences that envelop current social services practices.

The society within which professionals are expected to implement objective principles of aiding others has been increasingly contaminated by an individualistic, competitive ethos that, in a kind of Gresham's law, tends to drive out the fundamental values of community responsibility and cooperation. Privatization of services has strengthened competing motivations of profitable self-interest over community service, diminishing the traditional and structural safeguards of voluntary and public agency standards. Designed to use community resources to meet the deficiencies of societal institutions, social services have been chronically underfinanced simply as a stopgap adjunct to the economic market thus forcing organizational and functional compromises that impede sound practices and compound ethical problems.

As social workers have demonstrated their professional competency, they have been recruited into all societal institutions in the United States to aid people in dealing with fundamental systems. Consequently, new and different value conflicts arise, requiring the translation of professional responsibility into uncharted fields. New technology, research and increased specialization of practice have intensified knowledge and skill requirements that alter the levels and standards of professional practice. Computers, employee assistance programs in industry, and permutations of practice techniques have put the application of values to severe tests. These challenges are not new to the social work profession: it has a history of developing services for the caring components of a seemingly uncaring society. Developing services seem to have intensified as social workers have become more of an integral requirement for the maintenance of society.

Professional social workers, functioning in this maelstrom of contradictory stated and practiced values, have struggled to distill from the reality of their practice those principles and accompanying behaviors which will give strength to those whose lives are distortions of the human spirit, mind, and body.

As Jane Addams muses in her book *The Excellent Becomes the Permanent*, "Ideals are 'true' in the definition of William James in that they have been 'assimilated, validated, corroborated, and verified in experience,' that they are fruits of life." The ideals of social work practice — those fruits of life — have had a lifelong cultivator in Charles Levy, whose thinking, teaching, and writing has been primary in clarifying the semantics of values, ethics, and ethical behavior.

Levy guided his Task Force colleagues through the labyrinth of preferences, conflicting experiences and traditions to produce the NASW Code of Ethics which, when combined with the International Federation of Social Workers Code of Ethics, has been the standard for ethical practice for many years. Now, he increases the debt of all of us to him for his full explication of the premises of social work ethics and their application. As a practitioner who has had to deal with ethical issues in every aspect and level of social work practice, I have found a great sense of security in Levy's delineation of the genesis, purpose, limitations, and scope of social work ethics in this publication. I hope it will become a standard for the integration of values and ethical behavior into social work education, as well as a guidebook for agencies and individual practitioners. Its title might well have been *The Encyclopedia of Social Work Ethics*.

Chauncey A. Alexander, ACSW, CAE

Chapter I

The Many Splendored Sphere of Ethics

ETHICS AS VALUED CONDUCT

Ethics are the application of values to human relationships and transactions. Whatever the substance of exchanges between persons in personal, business, and professional relationships—whatever words, deeds, or material things pass between them—there are also understandings and expectations regarding the attitudes and behavior that are valued in the process. To the extent that these understandings and expectations guide and influence human relationships (and serve as a basis for evaluating human conduct), they represent the ethics of them.

Ethics regulate and control the behavior of participants in human relationships and transactions. In some situations ethics are more effective than in others, depending on the relationship between the participants; the transaction in which they are engaged; and the interest, influence, and authority of others in relation to both.

Although two friends may be concerned about, and even take seriously, others' reactions to what transpires between them, they are generally accountable to no one but each other for what they do or how they do it, unless, of course, laws are broken or actionable damage is inflicted in the process. If one friend, for example, promises the other to keep a secret and fails to do so, the result may be mutual alienation and perhaps disappointment and derogation, but rarely anything more serious.

However, a psychiatrist's revelation of the confidences of a patient, without the patient's permission or supportable justification, subjects the psychiatrist to penalties ranging from censure to deprivation of the right to practice. In each of the above cases the revelations may be considered unethical as long as keeping confidences is

1

valued. The different effects are due to the nature of both the relationship and the transaction between the participants.

VALUES AND ETHICS

Values are essentially preferences, and ethics are preferences that affect behavior in human relationships. They may be the preferences of the participants in those relationships. Or they may be the preferences of others with interest in, and perhaps a degree of authority over, what goes on in them.

There are all kinds of preferences, some less consequential and more innocuous than others. Preferences that are simply a matter of individual or group taste are relatively arbitrary. Although tastes (according to the Latin maxim) are not supposed to be arguable, they are often argued about, sometimes vigorously and aggressively. Tastes in food, drink, music, art, and drama are argued. Often, those with one preference will not comprehend the preference of others. Individuals and groups feel so strongly about their preferences that it affects their attitudes and behavior towards others who do not share those preferences.

Unless religiously, ideologically, politically, or culturally reinforced, preferences in food, music, literature, art, charitable giving, and ideas are generally matters of individual or group choice. Their intensity varies widely and changes over time and in response to experience. Tolerance of differences varies as well, certainly between national and group cultures, but also within nations and groups. Ethics tend to be less variable although they, too, are subject to change. Conformity, moreover, is hardly universal.

Disagreement, difference, dissent, deviation, and ambiguity notwithstanding, the conduct valued in human relationships and transactions is left less to individual and group discretion than other types of preferences. For such types as well, biases and prejudices often lead to assault, deprivation, and discrimination against those who differ. Since these behaviors also involve the way in which some persons are treated by those with opportunity to put them at a physical, social, emotional, or economic disadvantage, they fit the perspective of ethics that guides this discussion.

VARIETIES OF ETHICS

Values associated with the duties and obligations of participants in human relationships and transactions are the result of group consent and consensus. These values are subject to myriad influences, both historical and philosophical; they also reflect the biases and concerns of those who promote and promulgate them.

Whatever the theoretical influences on the formulation and selection of values, practical ethics requires an appreciation of human relationships and transactions as well as the duties and obligations incurred by the participants.

Some of these duties and obligations inhere in the substance of the exchange. One undertakes to do a job or perform a service for the other in exchange for an agreed-upon fee. That is the substance of the exchange between them. Ethics represent the framework of values that guide and constrain the participants during the job or service. A plumber, for example, expects to have the access necessary for getting the job done; the customer is expected to pay for it. The customer, in turn, expects the plumber to do the job, and to do it properly. These are understandings and values that, aside from allowing everything to be done that needs to be done in a society, permit a society to function smoothly and fairly. These are the kinds of values that participants in human relationships and transactions are expected to live by as they attend to their undertakings in relation to one another.

At the Level of Society and Government

Varieties of ethics may be distinguished by the level at which the relevant ethics operate, whether as phenomenon or expectation. Society is one of the more inclusive levels of relationship at which ethics operate to impose value-based expectations on participants. Society and government have duties and obligations toward their constituents, and constituents have reciprocal duties and obligations. Some are legislated; some are implied; some are inferred. Whether enforced by police powers or social pressures, these duties and obligations are presumably designed to ensure domestic tranquility and provide for the general welfare.

Duties and obligations of society and government toward constituents, and vice versa, define the responsibility each has in relation to the other. Government provides national security, public highways, health care, etc.; constituents provide taxes, obedience to the law, voting, etc. But duties and obligations go beyond the structure, means, and resources to fulfill the responsibility. Society and government declare the values to which they are committed, and those to which constituents are committed. Constituents are not (supposed to be) abused or treated arbitrarily by society and government. Nor do they cheat on taxes or bear false witness in court. Society and government encourage constituents to treat one another fairly, and induce a collective concern for the poor, the weak, the disabled, and the disadvantaged. Both society and government exercise courtesy and constraint when dealing with constituents. And both expect constituents to exercise courtesy and constraint in relation to one another. At least, that is what they are supposed to value in the fulfillment of their mutual duties and obligations.

Public and social policies are the vehicles through which those societal values are articulated that affect constituents and others. They reflect the ethics of society and government. They define expectations, and they guide their realization.

At the level of society and government ethics are often controversial. They are subject to the preferences of partisan politics and ideologies that sometimes defy consensus or resolution when they conflict. Decisions are made, however. Laws are passed. Courts deliver opinions. Principles are enunciated in public, social, and political arenas. With variable impact, depending upon the locus and authority of policies and their durability, values guide, if not govern, the various spheres of social and political life, even as dissent and debate persevere. Those values also guide and govern what society and government do. As such, they represent the ethics by which they and their constituents are guided and governed.

Within the array of social and public policies that reflect the ethics of society and government — aside from those that affect daily transactions with constituents and others — are policies that contend with some of the most troublesome and divisive value issues of our time. Because of reactions, when resolutions of those issues are indeed found, as in Supreme Court decisions, they often remain tenuous at best. Nevertheless, as decisions or the preponderance of views, they are the ethics of the moment, and represent conduct to be valued.

Conduct valued or disvalued in this category affects the removal of life supports; abortion; organ transplanting based on controversial definitions of death; the right to privacy; isolation of persons with AIDS; unconditional assistance to those in need of income, food, and shelter, etc.

Society's duties and obligations toward its constituents and others are expressed through preponderantly shared values and social pressures; those of government through legislative and administrative actions and through judicial decisions. Whether through encouragement of voluntary measures or enunciation of compulsory expectations, means and resources are provided that contribute to the health and welfare of constituents and others. The United States, for example, makes budgetary provision for emergency assistance to populations in states and nations afflicted by drought, flood, famine, and earthquakes.

Through volunteer and government organizations and procedures, provision is also made to safeguard the well-being of persons threatened by disease, by restricting the freedom of infected persons and providing, if not requiring, inoculation and quarantine. In addition, police and popular intervention forestalls or stops violence and the abuse of victims. In each of these cases, values are implied in both the objectives and conduct of society and government.

Even when an objective is clear and widely valued as societally and governmentally obligatory — what is "owed" on the part of society and government to constituents and others as part of their relationship and their mutual responsibility — other contravening values intrude to inhibit or postpone action. How effectively depends on the effectiveness of the dissent. Mass inoculation, quarantine, or testing sometimes proves sufficiently controversial, despite the clear and present danger of an epidemic, to generate disruptive resistance. Some people value their own privacy and prerogatives more than they do what is purported to be the general welfare. These people are sometimes successful enough to change a societal or government value and to redefine ethical responsibility. At the moment, for example, the isolation of persons with AIDS is vigorously decried in some quarters. At the same time, others insist on it, exempting no one, including children who crave the opportunity to be educated alongside their peers. Feelings are strong despite some doubt about how contagious or how transmissible the disease is. An ironic turn to the separate but equal concept of education, discredited in 1954, was taken in one elementary school in which the only concession made to one child infected with AIDS was to cage her in a glass booth in a classroom.

The valuation of the general welfare is also not sufficient to overcome the revulsion experienced in response to experimentation with human beings that endangers them (perhaps fatally), or simply deprives them of needed service or treatment. This, despite the scientific objective of finding a cure for a devastating disease. This is particularly true if the experiment is done without knowledge or consent. Such experimentation, despite its benevolent and humane intent and potential contribution to science and medicine, conflicts with conduct valued in relation to those adversely and unfairly affected.

At the Level of Social Organizations and Agencies

As entities, social organizations and agencies carry ethical responsibility as well. They, too, enunciate policies that represent what they value to be done in their relationships with members, patients, and clients, and what they value in the way it is done. What they are chartered, created, or otherwise undertake to do, they commit themselves to do. They incur the responsibility to do it. They assume, or are charged with, the responsibility to protect children, provide health care, provide counsel, make social and recreational opportunities available, and so on. This is the work that they are established and sanctioned, by law or communal accord and support, to do. However, the consideration, concern, courtesy, respect, and regard with which they do their work, and the conscientiousness and accountability with which they acquire and employ the personal and material resources for doing it, represent their ethics. On one hand, their ethics are a function of their relationship and responsibility to those they serve or represent; on the other hand, they are a function of their relationship and responsibility to their community and society.

Organizations and agencies, as such, obviously do not act. The people in them — and those who represent and work for them — act. The policies of the organizations and agencies, their ethical commitments, become the commitments of their personnel and leadership. These commitments become what others expect of them by way of valued conduct. Upon them devolves the ethical responsibility articulated or implicit in organization and agency purposes and policies. This includes responsibility to members, patients, and clients as well as community and society. It also includes the ethical responsibility of personnel and leadership to one another. The ethical responsibility assumed by and attributed to individuals who, separately or collectively, act in and for organizations and agencies is of the same order as that of other personal and occupational relationships. The difference is that the former is incurred by individuals in their capacities as representatives of organizations and agencies and as implementers of organization and agency purposes and policies.

Providing the programs and services of organizations and agencies in a competent, humane, respectful, and considerate fashion (and without bias, prejudice, or discrimination) is a prime requisite of those organizations' ethics. As for their ethical responsibility to their communities and to society, it is reflected in *whether* they do in fact address the purposes for which they exist, and observe the policies they enunciate. It is also reflected in the honesty, economy, and integrity with which money, facilities, equipment, personnel, and other resources are employed, and in their relevance to the purposes for which they are intended.

Whether acting for, and on behalf of, organizations and agencies or society and government, the ethics of individuals affect *whether* they attend to their tasks as well as *how*. The payment and acceptance of bribes in the awarding of defense and other types of contracts affects the relative fairness of the bidding for and awarding of contracts. It also affects the quality and cost of the contracts. Similarly, the extortion of bribes by health and safety inspectors affects the fairness with which inspections are done. It also induces neglect of the function which the inspectors are assigned — with detrimental personal and physical consequences for consumers and personnel. Comparable effects are likely in organizations and agencies when duty is similarly neglected or compromised.

At the Level of Occupational Groups

Occupational groups and professions carry ethical responsibility as identifiable and responsible entities. Because of their status and functions in society, they often assert, or have ascribed to them, what they value for their members, for people in general, and for those they serve or with whom they do business. Through the circulation or codification of the ethics to which they as groups, subscribe, they publicly declare the ethics to which they and their members collectively are said to be committed, and the ethics that others may confidently expect of them.

Admittedly, it is difficult to conceive of an unethical conduct charge against an occupation or profession as a whole, but occupations and professions are usually concerned enough about their collective standing and their credibility to be sensitive to any criticism that they are not living up to expectations. Moreover, what is assumed as a collective commitment of a group, is sometimes expressed — through a code of ethics, for example — as a requirement for each of its members. The expectation that lawyers will do pro bono work is a case in point, although enforcement is sometimes unwieldy. Consensus regarding its acceptance is not always easy to come by either, despite extensive acknowledgement of its appropriateness as valued conduct befitting the ethics of a learned profession.

At the Level of Individual Actors and Actions

Ethics define the duties and obligations of participants in relationships and transactions associated with the performance of occupational and other roles. The nature and context of the relationships and transactions will determine the extent and direction of ethical responsibility. It will tend to be reciprocal in simple transactions like those in which goods are bought and sold. Barring deviation from common standards, the terms of exchange between buyer and seller will be comparable in value. Hence ethical responsibility will be shared fairly equally: so much money for so many goods. The goods will be as represented, and the check in payment will not bounce. At least these will be the valued behaviors, and therefore the mutual expectations. Professional relationships and transactions—those in which informed, skilled, and sensitive service is provided—tend to be less simple and require differentiated ethical responsibility between the participants.

The ethical responsibility in each case is that of an individual in the performance of an assigned or assumed role. Thus, society may or may not value the removal of the life supports sustaining a patient in an enduring and irreversible coma. The basis for evaluating ethical judgment, however, is what a specific physician or nurse does, or is expected to do, in fulfillment of a professional responsibility to a specific patient because of an acknowledged professional relationship. There may, of course, be other claims on the actor's accountability (e.g., the law or societal preference), but ethical judgment in response to ethical responsibility is essentially an independent operation whatever the consequences of other requirements and influences.

Conduct that is valued by actors in human relationships and transactions, and by those who will react to their conduct, will be subject to differing appraisals, depending on the context and participants as well as other considerations and influences. However, in all situations to which ethical responsibility applies, the chief consideration is the responsiveness of actors to those duties and obligations that transcend the substance of the transactions between the participants.

FUNCTIONS OF ETHICS

Ethics serve a variety of purposes. A society is in fact virtually inconceivable without ethics, even a totalitarian society. In totalitarian societies, preferences and priorities govern the actions and relationships of constituents and the actions of societies and constituents in relation to one another, although many do not subscribe to those preferences and priorities and may be victimized by them.

In such societies, some behaviors are not only more valued than others, they are also subject to more severe penalties, with sanctions written into law (including criminal law). Collaboration by constituents in enforcement, moreover, is often credited and rewarded, the cruelty and arbitrariness of the consequences for innocent persons notwithstanding. A child who informs on parents, if they criticize the government, for example, earns governmental kudos. Loyalty to government exceeds filial duty in value. On the other hand, a child in the United States who "peached" on his addicted parents was congratulated. The difference was not that this act was considered ethical on its face, for loyalty to parents is still valued, but that the child was regarded as properly responsive to a higher value: the parents' and therefore the family's well-being.

Values vary from culture to culture, but they are relatively constant within cultures. At the least, they don't come and go randomly and spasmodically. Time and circumstances do have their impact, and counterforces persist with sometimes radical effects. Conservatives also persist, at times successfully enough to revive old values and reinstate, as a preponderant or operational view, preferences for behavior valued in the past. Social conditions, accumulated knowledge, modified attitudes, political conflict, social action, charismatic leadership—all contribute to changes, including reversal, at all levels of social structure and activity. The treatment of Afro-Americans in the United States before the Civil War was much different from their treatment after the war. And their treatment since the 1960s has been much different than it was before the 1960s, and not only because of legislation. Gaps remain nevertheless. The ethics of whites in relation to Afro-Americans, by and large, must still be regarded as changing, with some sites and spheres of activity manifesting more deficiencies than others. In some settings, and in some social roles, more is expected by way of valued conduct—sometimes demanded and required—than in others.

The same may be said of men in relation to women, and heterosexuals in relation to homosexuals, etc. The ethics of professions, on the other hand, while hardly a reflection of the uniform commitments of each member, have tended to be more stable. Perhaps this is because they have been codified, applied, enforced, and studied more consistently and systematically than ethics for persons and

societies at large. Still, the ethics of professions continue to be re-
vised and debated.

Whatever the nature and status of ethics in any society or seg-
ment of society (social, legal, occupational, and so on), and whatever the degree of their formalization, they have tended to perform
one or more of several functions. Some are phenomenological,
some ideological, and some regulatory. One of these is a normative
function.

As Norms

This is a phenomenological description. It identifies conduct that
has come to be valued over time in particular contexts. Provision
may very well be made for it by governments, organizations, occupations, cultural groups, and all kinds of informal groups, including
street corner gangs. It may be legislated, touted, implied, intimated, or understood. It may be codified or assumed. It represents
the way things are properly done, and done properly.

Depending upon the values of society and one's own values, as
well as one's inclination to live and act by them, restraint may be
exercised in dealing with others over whom one may have an unfair
advantage. Kicking a man when he is down is just "not done."
Seducing an inebriated adult is looked down upon.

For those, like social workers, with responsibility to others
within specifically defined and regulated relationships, the reaction
is less permissive. The test of deviation is also more demanding. A
person can get away with more in casual, informal, and family relationships than in professional relationships. Still, the values to
which actors are held, or to which they hold themselves in all relationships, constitute potent if variably effective constraints.

Normative values that govern behavior in human relationships
and transactions exist in the mind of the actor or the observer, usually both. They perpetrate an observable effect on either or both
without regard to possible sanctions. All are not equally committed
to those values, or guided by them, but they exist as social phenom-
ena of which there is considerable awareness.

As Aspirations

Another function of ethics, its aspiratory function, is of a rather different order. This function represents how some people in a society or group would like conduct to be within human relationships and transactions. Acts of loving kindness, as idealized in Judaic literature for example, cannot simply be legislated, but they are highly valued. Citizens and members of religious and ethnic groups cannot usually be forced to make charitable contributions to service organizations and persons in need. They are not subject to incarceration and other penalties if they fail to do so. However, in both secular and sectarian terms, our society values charity sufficiently to amount to intimidation for many. Analogically, members of professions are importuned — sometimes with enunciated and codified principles of ethics — to make themselves and their services available without cost to the poor and the deprived. Even when codified, and thus perceived and treated as obligatory if not enforceable expectations, such principles are often controversial in substance, degree, and implementation. Professional associations often experience difficulty obtaining acceptance of the principles and, when they succeed, often have difficulty effecting consistent conformity.

Although "doing good" for relatively vulnerable and deprived persons is generally regarded as ethical in our society, in the view of many it is better left to each person. It therefore remains, to a great extent, an aspiration rather than a phenomenon.

As Prescriptions

The prescriptive function of ethics makes ethics less voluntary. Expectations are defined for family and other relationships in which certain conduct is sufficiently valued to make deviation or neglect not only censurable but actionable. Penalties may be imposed by law or organizational procedures.

Though business is business in our capitalist country, and competition its life blood, insider trading in the stock market is verboten. Use of inside information and bribery in the quest for defense contracts is also forbidden. The use of drugs in athletic competition subjects offenders to serious consequences, whether the intent is recreational or to gain unfair advantage over competitors. What is prescribed is required, and what is required is often legislated by government or organization, sometimes both.

The full range of ethics' functions applies to all levels and loci of society, including its professions. Their operation varies from setting to setting depending on the nature of the activity, its status in society, the kinds of participants it involves, the nature of their relationships, their relative risks and advantages, and so on.

PREMISES OF ETHICS

Relative Positions of Actors

What is expected by way of valued conduct in formal or informal social settings (i.e., the principles of ethics by which persons are expected to be guided in their actions) derives from elements generally present in human relationships and transactions. One of these is the position of the actor, to whom expectations will be applied as they affect relationships to others, and the effects of the actor's conduct and responses on them. A salesperson who sells a necklace to an uninformed customer is ethically bound not to pass off brass as gold. This may very well be poor salesmanship. It may be impractical. Whatever else it may be, it is also unethical. A person who is in a position to know more than another, and to profit from the disparity of knowledge, and who then uses that disparity to hoodwink the other, is acting unethically. That is, providing that honesty in commercial transactions of this type is societally or occupationally valued, whether as a social and commercial norm or as a better business credo. In that light, it becomes a principle of ethics for the salesperson. And, in that light it becomes a reasonable expectation on the part of the customer.

Similarly, it is not cricket for a neighbor who has been entrusted with the key to a vacationer's apartment to burglarize that apartment. The possession of the key puts the neighbor in a position to violate the trust implicit in the transfer of the key. Doing so in contravention of the purpose for the transfer is therefore unethical. Again, this assumes the valuation of the trust.

The relationship between the parties in this case is less formal than in that of the necklace. It is not, as in the case of the necklace, an occupational relationship for which mutual obligations are more specifically defined and sanctioned. Of course, there are the criminal implications and consequences of the apartment burglary as such. In more general terms, the burglary is also an unethical act, however voluntary the responsibility assumed, and the absence of an explicit quid pro quo between the neighbors notwithstanding.

In a professional relationship the disparity of knowledge and opportunity between the participants is especially noteworthy, as in medicine, psychiatry, and social work. The position of the practitioner represents the a fortiori case of ethical responsibility. The relationship is both formal and sanctioned. It is also regulated. The responsibilities of the participants are scrupulously defined to reflect the different expectations applied to them.

The criteria used to evaluate the ethics of participants in all these cases are quite similar. However, their operation varies according to the nature of the activity in each case, the nature of the relationship and responsibility, the manner in which these are perceived and provided for in society, and so on. The values associated with the expectations are less affected than the intensity with which they are regarded and institutionally or legally provided for.

Relative Vulnerabilities of Actors

A critical premise of ethics and ethical responsibility is the opportunity of some persons to adversely affect others because of the differences in their positions or situations. To the extent that one person is weaker, less intelligent, more dependent, less capable of exercising judgment, or disadvantaged by another — and the latter's position or role makes it possible to exploit such deficits — does the latter accrue ethical responsibility. Physical or sexual child abuse is certainly unethical, whatever else it is, in our society. The theft or embezzlement of an incapacitated person's resources by a son, daughter, or attorney, is unethical, whatever else it is. Deprivation of a patient's access to available medical care by a physician is unethical. If such deprivation is justified on other grounds — even rational and compelling ones — it is still unethical, although a case might be made for superseding considerations. In each case the issue turns on the vulnerabilities of one participant as compared with another in a relationship.

Relative Risks for Actors

Whatever the setting and circumstances of human relationships and transactions, there are relative risks and hazards for one of the participants at the hands, or under the influence, of another. The issue posed for ethical judgment and resolution, as well as evaluation, is what one participant has to risk or lose in a relationship or transactions and the responsibility and opportunity the other has as a result. Whatever a person values — money, autonomy, access to goods and services, legal rights or representation, physical well-being, emotional stability — that is at risk because of a relationship or transaction and his or her relative position in it, becomes a premise of ethics and ethical responsibility when it is in real or potential jeopardy. If the value is a perverse or self-destructive one in the view of the other, it is no less a premise of ethics and ethical responsibility. What is different for the other is the nature of the ethical judgment to be made and of the action to be taken as a result.

One may value what one already has and is at risk of losing, or what one may not have but is seeking in a relationship or transaction (a job or education, for example). To the extent that someone else may be in a position to make it available, whether on justifiable or arbitrary grounds, that person's ethics are at issue. In prospect or actuality, whatever a person is at risk of being unjustly or unfairly deprived of in a human relationship or transaction constitutes a premise of ethics and a basis for the expectation of valued conduct.

Relative Opportunities for Actors

Whatever of value that anyone may be deprived of by another, represents an opportunity for the latter to exploit. The exploitation of the opportunity need not be aggressive, although it may be. One may value one's secrets and share them, in trust, with another. In professional relationships, such sharing may be a prerequisite for service. Whatever the circumstances, the possession of the secrets represents an opportunity to reveal them. Whether the secrets shared are those of a troubled patient or client, or of an employer in a competitive enterprise, each person has reason to expect the secrets to be held in confidence — again, this assumes the valuation of care and restraint.

Other opportunities are afforded to participants in human relationships and transactions, not the least of which is the very opportunity *not* to do what one is committed, or responsible to do. As such it, too, is a significant premise of ethics and ethical responsibility.

VIEWS OF ETHICS

In quotidian relationships and transactions, ethics range from that which is simply desirable, from the point of view of conduct that is valued, through that which is optimal for a society to function smoothly and morally, to that which is imperative if the society is to function at all.

No disaster is likely to occur if people are not entirely courteous, civil, and considerate, but relationships and transactions are apt to be more harmonious if they are. That is what makes such responses desirable. Competition is normal in our market economy, and optimal if fair and above board. Unduly ruthless competition, however, is not. In some contexts, expectations for valued conduct are so seriously regarded that they become imperative, sufficiently so that provision is made for their enforcement, if not through law or institutional procedures, then through the effectiveness of social and group pressures.

The practice of human service professions is one of those contexts although it, too, is governed by ethics that range from the desirable, through the optimal, to the imperative. Variations occur within and between professions as to which it may be, and the seriousness with which it is regarded and provided for. Variations also occur from time to time and from case to case, depending upon what is valued in its time, the participants' vulnerabilities and opportunities, the status and posture of the affected profession, and other variables.

Codes of professional ethics reflect the different intensities with which valued conduct may be regarded. Some principles of codified ethics suggest what may be desirable; some what may be optimal; and some what may be imperative.

Nevertheless, compared with ethics that govern personal and quotidian relationships and transactions, professional ethics (those that govern the conduct of practitioners in various professions) are more systematically and compellingly conceived. By no means do professional practitioners have exclusive and autonomous jurisdiction over their professional ethics, although they are allowed considerable discretion in making their ethical judgments. This is not without some degree of accountability, however. To whom they may be accountable varies from profession to profession. Some professions are authorized to bring the force of law and the courts to bear upon deviants (e.g., the legal profession). Others may be limited to the pressure of their professional associations and intimidation implicit in the threat of being dropped from association rolls. A practitioner's conduct that results in injury to others may, of course, subject the practitioner to the sanctions of law.

Chapter II

Premises of Social Work Ethics

Social work ethics guide, regulate, and control the behavior of social workers in their capacity, roles, and status as social workers. Social work ethics represent what is expected of social workers in the performance of their professional functions and in their conduct as members of the social work profession.

What is expected of social workers by way of valued conduct in their professional functions and status, is based upon and derives from the work that they do; those for whom, and with whom, they do that work; and the settings in which they do it.

The starting point of professional responsibility is quality of work and competence. Social workers are expected to be able to perform the functions they are assigned and those for which they assume responsibility. Aside from provision made for students and trainees to develop skills under the tutelage and supervision of qualified and experienced social workers, competence is an ethical prerequisite to undertaking the performance of social work functions.

Behaviors and attitudes valued in the actual performance of social work functions, from the initiation and maintenance of necessary relationships through all the transactions affecting their performance, describe the particulars of social work ethics. These include the principles and desiderata of social work ethics, and criteria for the appraisal of their application by social workers.

SOCIAL WORKERS AS FOCUS
OF ETHICAL RESPONSIBILITY

Although all participants in social work enterprises are expected to behave ethically, primary responsibility for ethical conduct — at

19

least as governed by codes of social work ethics—is attributable to, and required of, the social workers in them. Codified principles of social work ethics refer primarily to the values and ethical aspirations to which social workers are expected to be committed.

Clients with whom they work and others whom they affect in their practice and conduct are not entirely exempted from adherence to standards of ethical conduct, but the greater burden is imposed on the social workers.

One of the reasons is that social workers are the presumed activators of social work enterprises. They activate the processes through which purposes and goals may be realized when they assume or are assigned professional responsibility. Success is neither promised nor inevitable, but social workers are employed, or undertake (as private practitioners, for example) to make the attempt. They are presumed to have the requisite background and education to do so.

CONTENT AND CONTEXT
OF SOCIAL WORK ETHICS

The assumption of professional qualifications is a major premise of social work ethics. It is also a rationale for assigning social workers relatively greater ethical responsibility. In terms of social work knowledge and skill, the disparity between social workers and those they serve (as well as those they often affect) represents advantages and opportunities warranting differential expectations. Principles of social work ethics are designed to prevent social workers—or at least to discourage or deter them—from exploiting those they are supposed to serve or are in a professional position to affect.

The Possession and Use
of Social Work Competence

More affirmatively, and as such a positive premise of social work ethics, social workers, who are presumed and expected to have knowledge and skills that their clients do not possess, and to whom is assigned or ascribed professional responsibility in relation to them, are ethically bound to apply their knowledge and skill in their clients' interests. Clients, for one thing, resort to social workers to be served and not to be disserved. The interests of others who may be affected in the process must also be taken into account. However, these are not always accommodated if the interests of affected parties happen to conflict with one another and require choosing among them. The validity of such choices would have to be substantiated, however, on grounds of either professional or ethical responsibility, or both. Principles of social work ethics offer social workers guides and restraints in making such choices.

Relative Vulnerability of Clients

Another premise of social work ethics, and a reason for assigning relatively greater ethical responsibility to social workers, particularly in relation to clients, is the relative vulnerability of clients. This is certainly true of clients with pressing needs and problems of the sort that direct them to social workers for help. Clients in crisis, or in a state of despair for one reason or another, are likely to suffer impaired judgment and to become inordinately dependent upon the social workers. This situation requires added responsibility for scrupulously disciplined and restrained responses and actions. In such circumstances, the decisions and reactions of clients can be unduly influenced by their perceptions of the social workers' preferences, however distorted. Their decisions are not likely to be independently calculated choices of options for which they are practically and emotionally ready, if indeed they are serviceable for their needs at all.

Clients whose judgments are limited under any circumstance, by nature or immaturity, developmental deficiencies, or disability, are that much more likely to be at the mercy of social workers' discretion. This makes social work ethics all the more clearly imperative.

Risks for Clients

Implicit in these premises of social work ethics (and in relation to which guides and principles are essential) is still another premise: the risks to which clients are exposed in the very act of resorting to social workers for help. One of the risks for clients is sheer discovery— public awareness of the fact—which they may have reason to keep secret.

More substantively, another risk for clients is the social worker's neglect of the need or problem that caused clients to seek service. The neglect may be due to refusal of the service or to negligence or incompetence once service is undertaken. Clients in treatment also risk the loss of whatever is of tangible or intangible value to them. They can be deprived of anything and everything from their self-esteem to their fortune.

One circumstantial reason for the reliance on social workers' ethics is the risk inherent in the reality that the practice of social workers is not commonly observed by others. In fact, some of the principles applicable to the functions of social workers require privacy as a matter of both practice efficacy and professional ethics. To speak and act freely and without fear or reservation, in order to be well served, and to avoid embarrassment and unwanted exposure, clients are presumed to need and to be entitled to the shelter and assurance of privacy.

This may be as true for groups of clients as for individual clients, whether the groups are families or social, self-help, or clinical groups in which they are helped with needs and problems they experience individually and collectively.

VARIATIONS IN EXPECTATIONS BASED ON SOCIAL WORK ROLES, RELATIONSHIPS, AND RESPONSIBILITIES

Although all human service professions share premises and principles of ethics, there are differences among them in terms of the risks for clients and the opportunities practitioners have for deviation. These are associated with the kind of work that is done and those for whom it is done. That is, it matters not only who they are, as far as age, sex, and mental and physical capacity are concerned, but also the circumstances and conditions that bring them to the attention of professional practitioners.

Social work ethics do differ in some respects from the ethics of other human service professions because of the kind of work social workers do, the kind of people they do it with, the kinds of reasons for which they do it, and the circumstances under which they do it. There are also differences within the social work profession, for which social work ethics must make provision, because of the range and diversity of roles that social workers play, the responsibilities that they carry, and the relationships they engage in with clients and others as a result.

Even when social workers perform similar professional roles and carry similar responsibilities, clients and circumstances vary sufficiently to require, if not fundamental differences in principles of ethics, then differences in their application. These are not simple variations that emerge from day-to-day or moment-to-moment changes that take place in all types of social work practice. Rather they are basic differences due to the nature of the roles, relationships, and clienteles of social workers. A review of some diverse roles that social workers perform in their practice should make this quite evident.

Clinical Social Work

Clinical social work may be defined as social work practice affecting clienteles directly as individuals or as groups and oriented to their goals, needs, and problems. In each case, the focus is on individuals as individuals, groups as groups, or individuals within groups. The range of goals, needs, and problems addressed by clinical social workers stretches from serious, critical ones affecting the functioning and well-being of persons in a state of social or psychological despair, through the normal developmental impasses of age, sex, religion, and personal relationships, to straightforward opportunities for personal, social enrichment through educational, recreational, social, and other programs. The categories along this continuum of goals, needs, and problems are not discrete but overlap and intermingle because neither clients nor vehicles of service fit neatly into any one of the categories at any one time or stage.

At one extreme, persons who seek, or who are referred for, social work treatment and service may be in a very fragile mental or emotional state. They are in particular need of the protection of social work ethics, whether social workers provide for them in their practice, or professional associations, institutions, or government agencies monitor and enforce them. Persons in such a state may not be in sufficient possession of their faculties to safeguard their rights and prerogatives. They may be excessively compliant and suggestible. A particular order of discipline, restraint, and discrimination is therefore required by social workers in the use of their influence.

Other persons in clinical social work treatment may not be especially vulnerable or deficient in their faculties, but may nevertheless be afflicted with feelings and inadequacies that deprive them of the will and judgment they would otherwise have. Out of gratitude to their social workers for the care and concern they are shown, and out of dependency, they may be inclined to let their guards down. In such circumstances, the constraints of social work ethics are needed, if not to shelter them from the idiosyncracies and inclinations of social workers, then to ensure the quality of treatment and service they require and deserve, even if they are not entirely alert to shortcomings.

In clinical social work, some persons being provided developmental and social opportunities lack neither poise nor capacity in their personal or social functioning. For them, the shelter and protection of social work ethics is not required so much as an optimal level of honesty, effort, civility, respect, and attention to tasks at hand on the part of social workers in the implementation of their professional responsibilities.

These, in fact, constitute the conduct valued for clinical social workers in the performance of their professional functions, whether clients are socially disabled or extremely competent. These social workers are accountable for such conduct as they apply their professional skills and knowledge in the service of their clients, from the beginning to the end of their professional relationships.

Community Social Work

A somewhat different order of direct service provided by social workers is that to community organizations. These may be grass roots or neighborhood organizations concerned primarily or exclusively with shared problems and goals — local conditions and services, inadequate or insufficient housing, homelessness, drug dealing, and so on — or with general needs and interests for which residents of a particular area plan and solicit support. Or they may be more complex and broadly based fundraising, planning, and coordinating organizations that support facilities and services for large population groups composed of persons who reside in a defined geographic area (e.g., regional or national) or who share ethnic, religious, racial, national, or other identifications for the purpose of advancing common interests and goals.

Community organizations vary in size, scope, funding, influence, and investment of time, energy, and resources by those who participate in them and manage them. The size and structure of organizational staffs also vary widely.

Social workers who staff the larger community organizations collaborate with other professional personnel who are charged with achieving organizational objectives, purposes, and goals. Depending upon their size, scope, functions, and relationship to their community, among other things, these staffs may include lawyers, accountants, public relations practitioners, and others. Social workers may also work with volunteer policy makers, fundraisers, planners, and others on boards, commissions, committees, and other structures. Within these, social workers apply their professional skill and knowledge. Within these, one finds applicability of social work ethics closely comparable to that in clinical social work because of contacts and relationships similar to those with social work clients.

However, social workers in community organizations are charged with implementing planning, fundraising, problem-solving, and other functions that community organizations perform, rather than providing personal services to those who participate in the work and administration of the organizations. The professional ethics by which they are guided, and to which they are committed, therefore affect their relationship with staff and volunteers in their capacities as participants in the organizations and not as clients in need of social work ministrations because of personal needs and problems.

Social workers are facilitators of the efforts of staff and volunteers on behalf of the organizations, but they are also concerned with their effects on staff and volunteers in the process. The professional values to which they subscribe, therefore, apply to those they deal with and to the organizations, although perhaps differently than they do to clients in treatment for needs and problems of their own. Basic principles of social work ethics do not vary so much from role to role as do the choice of principles that apply and how they are applied.

These differences are not negligible, however. For social workers to relate to community organization leaders as if they were clients, for example, by lapsing into a treatment mode, however manifest the need for treatment, is a confusion of both practice goals and ethics. It represents the misappropriation of a professional role at the expense of an assigned one, and it is therefore unethical.

This does not mean that community organization participants' need for treatment, when detected by social workers in the course of their practice, is ignored altogether. First, it is taken into account by social workers in the application of their social work skill and knowledge. Second, social workers have the ethical responsibility—through guidance, suggestion, referral, or other means suited to persons, situations, and circumstances—to help those in need of treatment to receive it.

Interorganizational and Interprofessional Social Work

Similar to social work in community organizations, and in fact often a component of social work in community organizations, is the work of social workers in organizations of organizations. Indeed, some organizations are organizations of organizations of organizations, whether of community organizations (as in the United Way and welfare councils) or of professional associations (as in the National Association of Social Workers before it became a single professional association of social workers).

Social workers who staff such multi-layered organizations are often two, three, or four steps removed from the ultimate constituents of such organizations, their individual members. This means that the social workers do not work with individuals, primary groups of such individuals, or, in many cases, even networks of such groups that are represented directly or indirectly in organizations of organizations of organizations. For example, a council of federations represents local federations which, in turn, represent local social agencies and community organizations, only some of which serve clients or have constituent or participating members. The internal structures of some social agencies and organizations may follow this same pattern (the B'nai B'rith or the National Association for the Advancement of Colored People, for example).

In the interprofessional sphere, organizations, whether permanent or transitory, represent professional associations that either share interests or goals or assemble to cope with issues and problems about which they share concern. Although they may start as ad hoc structures organized for action on those issues and problems, they sometimes find themselves dealing with additional issues and concerns and then evolve into more permanent structures.

The distance between social workers, who staff such interorganizational or interprofessional structures, and their ultimate consumers or constituents represents a premise of the professional ethics to which they are presumed to be committed. Though they may not deal directly with those consumers and constituents, they have an obligation (i.e., ethical responsibility) to them. The implementation of this duty is reflected in the way they relate to those with whom they do deal directly.

Social workers also have duties toward each of the constituent organizations with, or on behalf of which, they work, and the personnel and others who work for or represent them. Social work ethics, at least, require awareness of, and attention to, the interests of those who compose and are represented in those organizations. Such awareness and attention may also be conducive to effective social work practice and optimal use of social work skills and knowledge, but they certainly have ethical import and consequences.

As for ethical responsibility to those persons social workers work with directly and on a day-to-day basis in the fulfillment of professional responsibility and the performance of assigned functions, it corresponds closely to what has been described for social work in community organizations, again with differences in degree and professional intentions.

Supervision

Social workers who carry assigned responsibility for the supervision of other social workers and social work students are also subject to the expectations of social work ethics. Again, the principles of ethics social workers are presumed to be guided by, and committed to, do not coincide in all respects with those principles that guide and govern their relationships and work with clients and others whom they serve directly and in their own interest. On the contrary, the kinds of responses to duties to clients in treatment are likely to be misplaced with supervisees, whether paid staff or students, and with consequences antithetical to social work ethics if not to effective supervision.

Basic principles of social work ethics are nevertheless applicable, although they may be tempered or modulated for aptness to the purposes and ends of supervision. Thus, for example, social workers do not authoritatively hold clients to prior and arbitrary standards of achievement in relation to the needs and problems that are the substance of their exchange and interactions. The exceptions, of course, are those very selective pre-conditions of service that are set, (for example, for alcoholics and drug addicts) and which are part and parcel of the treatment process. Social workers do help and encourage other clients to aim for the achievement of their treatment goals.

Social work supervisors, on the other hand, must hold social work supervisees and students to standards of professional achievement. It is their assigned mission to do so, for professional employees as a matter of adequate job performance, and for students as a matter of systematic gate-keeping for the social work profession. An ethically as well as professionally calculated helping process is included to make success and development possible for both.

Social work supervisors hold professional employees to job expectations while making it possible for them to meet those expectations. As for social work students, supervisors have the duty to provide opportunities for them to acquire the knowledge and develop the skill necessary for entry into the social work profession, with the assurance of prospects for ethical and competent social work practice. A primary concern in the supervision of both staff and students is the effect on actual and prospective clients.

It is neither practical nor ethical for social work supervisors to deal with staff on the same terms as students. Staff are assumed to be able to perform assigned functions, given a modicum of administrative and supervisory support and a reasonable opportunity to succeed. On the other hand, students must have opportunities to learn what they need to know, and to acquire the skills they need to have for careers as social workers, assuming the necessary oversight and monitoring exist to prevent injury to clients.

Social work ethics become imperative in light of the power implied in the supervisory function. Social work supervisors can have considerable control over the opportunities of staff for success and progress as employees, and over the access of students to professional careers. If they are to ensure fairness and equity for supervisees, social work supervisors need awareness (and the guidance and influence) of social work ethics as they confer and interact with supervisees; as they represent employing institutions to supervisees and vice versa; as they evaluate the performance of supervisees; and as they participate in other administrative processes and procedures that affect the opportunities, prospects, progress, and future of supervisees. Fairness and equity for supervisees does not imply any penalty or disadvantage for clients with whom supervisees work, whether as students or as staff, or any penalty or disadvantage to employing institutions. To both, social work supervisors retain accountability and ethical responsibility.

Administration

Social workers who manage social agencies, organizations, and institutions contend with issues that differ appreciably from those that emerge in direct service to individuals, groups, and communities. The distinction is not always very sharp, since they also invariably work with administrative groups of staff and volunteers. Thus they have direct contact and professional relationships with groups of individuals. Social work ethics of the type that applies to direct services are approximately relevant to these, if not exactly as to direct services to clients with problems, then as to groups engaged in common endeavors like those in community organizations. In such organizations, moreover, administrative processes and procedures are required for organizational management. Social workers who carry managerial along with other responsibilities have ethical responsibility applicable to administration as well.

The principles and application of social work ethics will therefore vary in relation to the particular role and situation, although not in the fundamentals to which all social workers are bound in all of their roles. Differences will affect the particular principles that apply, to what and to whom they apply, as well as the manner in which they are applied.

Suffice it to say that social workers in management positions, or with managerial responsibility, often have at their disposal (if not at their command) the material, financial, and personal resources of their employing organizations and institutions. Social work ethics are required to ensure economy, honesty, accountability, and restraint in the use and management of those resources. Social workers with managerial responsibility usually stand between their employing organizations and the community that supports them, and to which they are accountable as chartered trustees. Therefore, social work ethics apply to the manner in which the social workers represent those organizations in and to the community, and relate to it.

Social Work Education

The premises of ethics for social work educators are, in a number of respects, similar to those for social workers who supervise social work students. Social work educators—those with primarily academic and classroom responsibilities—are also in a position to wield power over social work students, and to affect their fate and their future. There are differences between them, however, that introduce students' exposures and vulnerabilities for which provision in social work ethics is essential.

Analogous to the ethical responsibility of supervisors to social work students is the expectation that social work educators be willing and able to provide academic opportunities to help students acquire knowledge and develop competence for entry into the profession as ethical social workers. Social work educators are also expected to pass fair, accurate, and independent judgment on students in order to meet their ethical responsibility to prospective clients and employers of students as well as others whom students may affect in their professional capacity and status.

Social work educators also have ethical responsibility to the educational institutions of which they are a part. They share the institutions' responsibility for the effective implementation of the educational mission of professional schools to select and equip students for competent and ethical social work practice.

When social work educators serve as liaisons to agencies and organizations in which students are placed for field instruction (i.e., for supervised field practice), the possibility of collusion, whether intentional or inadvertent, with either students or their supervisors, requires particular restraint and self-discipline. Ambiguities and alignments must be avoided so that educational opportunities are carefully and responsibly planned and provided, performance is systematically and sensitively evaluated, and educational expectations are met by all of the participants in the process. As liaisons, advisors to students, classroom instructors, and collaborators with school colleagues, social work educators must keep in mind the stakes of schools, agencies, students, community, clients and the social work profession in the outcome of social work education. Educators must provide for them in the competent and ethical performance of their various and complex roles, not excluding their roles as scholars and researchers.

Social Work Research and Scholarship

Social work educators and other social workers who conduct research and scholarly inquiries are presumed to be committed to the standards, conventions, and ethics of those activities. Misleading and fraudulent efforts can cause errors and great harm when they are used as a basis for further inquiry or service. They may also be used as a basis of unwarranted or undeserved rewards and advancement.

Social work ethics are also necessary to prevent the exploitation of assistants in the pursuit of inquiries, and the failure to acknowledge their contributions. This is especially true when it is done by social workers with the kind of power and authority that teachers, supervisors, and employers have over students and subordinates.

Myriad other hazards and offenses are possible in relation to research and scholarship, like plagiarizing, revealing the confidences of subjects and participants without their consent, or distorting the data acquired from their participation. Social work ethics also provide for the harm that can come to participants during inquiries of a hazardous nature about which participants are either not informed or misinformed, if indeed there is doubt about the ethics of conducting such inquiries at all.

Consultation

Social workers are often employed as consultants to agencies, organizations, institutions, businesses, social work departments, and other social workers. Since their services are presumably sought because of some felt need (e.g., help with a task or problem for which the consultees do not feel entirely equipped), reliance on social workers, and the prospect of damaging effects due to misplaced or ill-advised confidence in them, require the constraints of social work ethics. Consultees' pathology or extreme vulnerability need not be implied to make ethical conduct imperative for social work consultants. Sometimes the quest of consultees is for the kind of enriched understanding and honing of skills that may be possible with intervention and stimulation by a reputable and objective outside expert. The emphasis of social work ethics may be less on the protection of consultees than on behavioral expectations for consultants and directed toward conscientious and responsible performance.

Under the pressure of expectations and the pressure to demonstrate their own expertise, not to mention the pressure to validate consultation fees and the promise of future ones, social work consultants may venture observations and solutions that are neither timely nor suited to the task or problem posed by consultees. In such circumstances, the practical purposes of consultation may be no better served than the principles of social work ethics applicable to them. However, the failure of social work consultants to respond to situations as they actually exist, independently of their private agendas, poses issues for which the guidance and restraints of ethics are necessary.

SOCIAL WORK ETHICS BEYOND CLIENTS

The label *clients* implies relationships between social workers and those to whom they provide service, and with whom they practice what has been described as clinical social work. The term is not entirely felicitous because it implies a pathology which does not always characterize the state or need of clients. The term is meant, however, to suggest that the focus of social work attention is on what clients seek as individuals, families, or groups by way of help with needs and problems or recreational, educational, and developmental opportunities. In each case, social workers are working for the clients. Nevertheless, they may have concurrent ethical responsibility to others for a number of reasons: because of effects of work with the clients; because of legitimate, or even legal interest, in the clients; because of their stake in the fate, conduct, experience, and future of the clients.

Among those whose interests social workers may have to take into account and consider, as they choose their courses of professional conduct with clients, may be parents of minors; employers (their own and those of clients); insurers who pay the fees for service to the clients; and, ultimately, even communities and society which may bear the consequences of what clients do and what happens to them.

This does not mean that the interests of third parties, as they may be called, are invariably accorded higher priority than those of clients. On the contrary, social workers usually must have unequivocal reasons to justify a denial of priority to clients. This is certainly true in clinical social work, although unequivocal reasons are often hard to come by. Social work ethics, on the other hand, require contention with them. At any rate, it is clear that social work ethics do not stop at the border of the relationship between social workers and their clients.

SOCIAL WORKERS AND SOCIETY

Whether as a function of their work with clients or independently of it, social workers, as members of their profession, are ascribed ethical responsibility in relation to the collective interests of community and society. Whether enforceable or not, this responsibility implies efforts on behalf of those in need in the community and society as well as those whose rights and prerogatives are compromised or jeopardized.

Sometimes the job descriptions of social workers include responsibility for such efforts, whether as a primary assignment or a supplement to service to clients. Social workers may work in an organization whose function is to promote services to elderly persons, or they may work directly with elderly clients and, as a component of that work, engage in social action and advocacy for services to all elderly persons, their clients included. But even in the absence of specifically assigned functions, or specifically implied responsibility, social workers may have ethical responsibility for efforts in the public interest, and in the interest of those in the community and society who are in any way deprived or disadvantaged.

One of the media through which social workers can affect the general welfare, and for which they may share ethical responsibility, is that of public and social policy. This may be the result of a specifically assigned professional responsibility, because of the chartered functions of their agencies, for example. Or it may be an implied responsibility resulting from their membership in professional associations that undertake such activities as a component of their collective social responsibility. In both cases the objective would be to advance or influence communal and governmental policies that affect the needs or entitlements of general or particular populations and services to them.

EFFECT OF MULTIPLE PROFESSIONAL ROLES ON SOCIAL WORK ETHICS

Other social work roles may be identified. Whether assigned in specific jobs or implied because of membership in the social work profession, variations in the functions of social workers occasion variations in ethical responsibility (if not in the principles of ethics, then in the mode of their application). The selection of principles and the manner of their application in specific situations are affected by the kinds and number of roles performed by social workers in those situations, and the responsibilities and relationships affected or implicated in them. A social work supervisor confronting a supervisee may have to draw on principles of ethics relevant not only to supervision but to administration and service to clients. He or she must select some at the expense of others, depending on the interest and the roles to which priority is assigned when they conflict with one another. The manner in which these, in turn, are applied is often as much a matter of skill as ethics, since provision is required for ethical responsibility that may be neglected in relation to some persons and interests because of priority given to others.

SIGNIFICANCE OF SETTING
FOR SOCIAL WORK ETHICS

Along with the other variables that influence (or should) the choice of principles to be applied in any situation, and the manner of their application, must be included the type of setting in which social work is practiced. Setting is often associated with characteristics and circumstances that make clients dependent, vulnerable, and disadvantaged. Some settings should immediately alert social workers to risks for clients and themselves, for which their ethics must provide.

Clients of community centers and neighborhood houses who come and go freely and voluntarily, and who are free to accept or reject recreational and educational opportunities, may be subject to the influence and preferences of social workers who work with them, but they are still likely to have relative control over their choices. The more able and mobile they are, and the greater their access to other opportunities and settings, the more autonomous they are likely to be, however much they may value and use the suggestions, guidance, and counsel of social workers. This hardly makes social work ethics irrelevant, but it does put such clients less at the mercy of unethical social workers.

On the other hand, clients in mental hospitals and nursing homes, whose lives, activities, and access to resources and contacts are controlled by others, are far less autonomous and much more dependent on others, including social workers. The more disabled the clients, mentally or physically, the less autonomous and more dependent they are. Given a modicum of awareness, and limited contact with relatives or friends, they are also likely to fear deprivation and retribution by their caretakers. Social workers who work with them carry the preponderant, if not the entire, weight of ethical responsibility as compared with social workers who work with competent and resourceful clients better able to monitor and evaluate their ethics.

Inmates of correctional institutions may not suffer physical or mental impairments, but as punitively incarcerated wards of the state, their options are severely restricted. Their daily lives are closely supervised, and their space for free movement and recourse to intervention on their behalf is very much limited. They may not even be free to refuse or resist social work treatment. Though they are often hardened, aggressive, menacing, and intimidating, social workers who work with them are still at an advantage over them. At times, social workers make the difference between continued confinement and liberty, or torment and reassurance about the state of their families.

In more traditional situations, setting is also a consequential factor for social work ethics. In private social work practice, for example, not only are there no observers but, unlike practice in agency and institutional settings, there is no apparent controlling authority. It is just the social worker and the client.

In employee assistance programs, for a different type of example, authority is very much present for both clients and social workers. From employee-clients' points of view, even when in treatment upon their own initiative rather than that of employers, there is possible risk to jobs and uncertainty about the loyalty of social workers. For social workers, there is the pressure of accountability to employers, but also the pressure of obligations to clients. Both perceive conflicts and ambiguities that must be taken into account as issues of ethics as well as practice. Who clients are, where they are served, and under whose auspices, shape the selection and application of principles of social work ethics as well as principles of social work practice, and the choice between them when they conflict. What serves the cause of practice — for the purpose of effective service to clients, for example — does not always serve the cause of ethics, and vice versa. The *best* thing to do in the service of clients is sometimes not the *right* thing to do in the service of professional ethics. An action taken to effect a prompt solution to a client's problems might also intrude on the client's self-determination. Whether or not it is taken will depend upon the priority accorded to the client's self-determination.

FUNCTIONS OF CODES
OF SOCIAL WORK ETHICS

Codes of social work ethics serve as guides to ethical social work practice, criteria for the evaluation of the ethics of actual practice, and bench marks for the enforcement of social work ethics and the adjudication of unethical conduct complaints. Professional associations of social workers construct and promote codes of ethics to provide guidance and inspiration to members, in recognition of the importance of codes to the status of professions in the community and society, and the stake in the professional conduct of their members. Deviations on the part of members taint a profession as a whole. Social work associations are also concerned about the effects of the behavior and actions of members on clients and others, and on the continuing credibility of the profession and effectiveness of its services and practice.

To be maximally serviceable to the great diversity and range of social work roles, relationships, risks, and responsibilities, the content of social work ethical codes can only be general in nature. Principles of social work ethics, to serve the purposes of guidance, education, and enforcement, must be general enough to meaningfully apply to the varieties of clients, situations, and circumstances in social work practice. And yet they must be amenable to reliable interpretation. Excessive specificity is impractical in that codes cannot very well provide for all the possible variations and eventualities in social work practice and responsibility; nor can all possible situations be anticipated. However, they cannot be so abstract as to defy application and interpretation. At the same time, principles of ethics cannot be so elastic as to make likely random application and interpretation to suit the limiting biases, preferences, motives, and idiosyncracies of practitioners, evaluators, and adjudicators with less than objective vested interests.

Since codified principles of ethics affect responsibilities that may conflict with one another (e.g., responsibility to children and to their parents) codes may appear to contain glaring inconsistencies. However, different principles apply to different responsibilities. Social workers who carry concurrently different responsibilities, or within any one of them have responsibility to or for different persons and interests, may find themselves drawing on one or more principles in response to each responsibility. This dictates the ordering of priorities when selecting and applying ethical principles according to primacy of responsibility, both in general and in specific situations.

AIMS OF CODES

Codified principles of social work ethics are not always of the same order. Some amount to aspirations, recommendations, or preferences. That is, they are not cast as obvious imperatives. Neither are they readily enforceable. They are nevertheless presented as clearly desirable (for example, the expectation that social workers will volunteer their services after natural disasters and catastrophes).

Some principles represent norms: behavior in a professional capacity or status that has come to be valued and, under some circumstances, enforceable, depending on such things as the fragility of clients or social workers' positions of special trust and reliance. Acceptance of clients and respect for their dignity are always expected of social workers, but deviation may not always be sufficiently evident or egregious to warrant or validate a complaint of unethical conduct. Abuse or discriminatory actions against clients, however, might justify complaint and sanctions.

Other principles of ethics are regarded as prescriptive and imperative standards of professional conduct, the neglect or violation of which subjects social workers to the sanctions of professional associations and perhaps law. Confidentiality is one of the more common of these but, as with other principles in this category, the offense of concern is that primarily made against clients. There are

others that may or may not affect clients, and still merit enforcement and sanctions (lying about one's credentials as a social
worker, for example).

Violations may be appraised on the basis of who is or might be
affected (a child as compared with an adult, for example). Violations may also be appraised on the basis of the circumstances to
determine, for example, whether or not enforcement of the expected standard of ethical conduct is appropriate. A very different
judgment would probably be made of social workers who pre-empt
the self-determination of a severely retarded child as compared with
an intelligent and competent adult.

In short, the interpretation of code content requires consideration of diverse variables, whether for the purpose (from the viewpoint of social workers) of making ethical judgments or (from the
viewpoint of professional associations) inspiring ethical conduct
and enforcing it.

DISTINCTION BETWEEN PROFESSIONAL
PRACTICE GOALS AND ETHICS
IN SOCIAL WORK PRACTICE

Criteria for the selection of principles of social work ethics, and
for the evaluation of decisions and actions taken as a result, differ
from criteria for the selection and implementation of actions taken
to achieve assigned or assumed professional objectives. Social
work ethics are consistent with the inalienable rights and prerogatives of those who are served by social workers and those who are
affected by their decisions and actions. These rights and prerogatives are made all the more inalienable by the risk of their denial as
a consequence of clients' need for help and their quest for it.

As a guide to social work actions and decisions, and as a basis for
evaluating them, social work ethics are concerned with what is morally valued for clients and others rather than what fulfills professional responsibility to them. Ethical practice may or may not coincide with effective practice. Optimally, it does, as when ensuring
and encouraging client self-determination encourages the development of client capacity for effective and salutary decision making.

Practice goals and ethical responsibility may conflict and may be mutually exclusive, as when clients exercise their right of choice and are on the verge of choosing a course of action contrary to goals they chose and in relation to which they have sought social work help. Social workers are compelled to choose between the right exercised and the option selected. In spite of their professional inclination to do what they consider best for clients (e.g., steering clients away from their misguided choice), social workers may find it necessary to give precedence to the ethical responsibility to respect the clients' right of self-determination. They may still use their professional skills to alert clients to the alternatives at their disposal, and to the probable consequences of each of them. Whatever the choice of clients in that event, social workers would prepare themselves and the clients to cope with its consequences, without saying "I-told-you-so." That, too, is ethical responsibility, but it also requires social work skill.

THE LAW AND SOCIAL WORK ETHICS

Conduct valued by law and conduct valued by social work ethics may not always coincide. For example, when testimony of social workers, which affects the confidences of their clients, is ordered in the interest of justice to defendants whose acquittal depends on the testimony. The demands of law may thus conflict with principles of social work ethics to which social workers are committed and to which they are expected to conform. The threat of incarceration, should they accord priority to their ethics over the law, could influence their response, but their self-interest could hardly be sufficient justification for neglecting their ethical responsibility to their clients, and confidentiality is a virtually sacrosanct principle of social work ethics.

The choice between incarceration and confidentiality is discomfiting, but that may be a burden that social work ethics impose, and one for which social workers must be prepared. The burden cannot simply be passed on to clients for whose protection confidentiality is primarily designed in the first place. It is not designed to protect social workers.

The choice between justice for defendants and confidentiality for clients perhaps poses a more agonizing dilemma for social workers whose social values incline them in both directions. But since it is clients with whom and for whom they work, within the context of a limiting professional ideology tailored to the dimensions and risks of the work, clients are entitled to, and prescriptively accorded, priority. Other measures must be taken by those with primary responsibility for the legislation and administration of justice to provide for defendants and judicial procedures. Here again, social workers are not exempt from the professional responsibility to suggest to clients the option of waiving their right to confidentiality by a waiver of privilege, to save the life of defendants, perhaps, if they are subject to capital punishment.

SUBSTANCE OF SOCIAL WORK ETHICS

As this discussion indicates, social work ethics encompass an extensive range of professionally valued rights, prerogatives, opportunities, and behavior. These are valued because they bear upon the practice and activity of social workers in their capacity and status as social workers, in the variety of roles they perform, and in their relationships during performance of those roles. In large measure social work ethics derive from the various circumstances and settings in which social workers perform their myriad roles.

Social work ethics are also influenced by society and its institutions and groups, public and private. The issues that they raise or by which they are confronted suggest, if not compel, principles of ethics, and expectations to which social workers may or may not be held. Thus, certain forms of advertising, which may once have been considered unprofessional or actually prohibited by codes of professional ethics, become legitimate as societal concern about restraint of trade overtakes professions.

And the proliferation of protests, debates, and litigation about AIDS, birth control, drugs, abortion, and the right to life, has generated expectations. Some of these have found their way into codes of professional ethics. This effect is especially observable in cases of discrimination affecting groups that, until quite recently, were not very widely regarded as a source of egalitarian concern (e.g., homosexuals, women, and disabled persons).

The social work profession, like other professions, has been affected by these issues and developments. It continues to be affected by them, not always in the same way, not always with its consent, and not always with consensus about them within the social work profession. Sometimes the experience of one profession influences another. The social work profession has felt the impact of others.

Failures and questions of ethics in government, politics, medicine, and law, have sensitized social workers to their own need for effective standards of ethical conduct. Perhaps social work experience has suggested aspirations for other professions. Ethics are very much in the air and seeping into the texture of social work as in other professions, causing it to add to and modify the subject matter of its ethics, and to introduce questions about its operation and application. Social work ethics, like the ethics of all professions, is in a constant state of flux, as are the mind set and preoccupations of social workers about it.

Some principles of social work ethics are more enforceable or enforced than others, although the violation of very few by social workers incurs dire consequences. The direst of these is little more than suspension from the professional association and publication of the offense, which is dire enough for some social workers. The result may be quite different, and more serious, if the violation runs afoul of the law, or if it leads to a cause of action for malpractice. Other than that, the threat of penalties may be less effective as a deterrent to unethical conduct than education, encouragement, and example.

The major focus of social work ethics is on the behavior of social workers in their professional capacity and status, beginning with their comportment. Principles of social work ethics in this category are related not so much to social workers' behavior as they perform their various professional roles (although they might be) as to their actions and stances as persons who are social workers, without regard to actual and existing professional relationships.

Comportment of Social Workers

Social workers are expected to not be dishonest; perpetrate fraud, deceptions, or misrepresentations; engage in any conduct that reflects adversely on their profession or in any way casts doubt on its credibility or reputation as a social function within society. They are held to this expectation without regard to whether its infringement occurs, or is evident, in actual professional relationships. Social workers, moreover, are expected to not condone, connive, or collaborate with violations of principles of social work ethics, whether for purposes of personal gain or not. Impairment of ability to perform professional functions by drug or alcohol use is, of course, frowned upon, but so is unruly and destructive behavior or other public displays that simply subject social workers and the social work profession to public ridicule and censure.

Social workers are also expected to not exaggerate or lie about their credentials, competencies, or status (e.g., as to whom they represent or with what authority) to prospective clients and employers or public media.

Social workers are not supposed to compromise the independence of their professional judgment, or in any way to appear to do so (by acquiring a financial or other personal interest in the outcomes of their professional practice with clients, for example). Social workers are not supposed to delegate responsibility to others that they are presumed to be carrying themselves.

Social workers are cautioned against responding to clients and others in a manner that distorts their professional relationships or otherwise intrudes on their ability and opportunity to exercise optimal professional judgment, and to make optimal use of their professional skills in serving and working with clients. Integrity and objectivity are highly valued in these connections, both in their own right and as they affect others.

Social Workers and Their Clients

The responsibility to clients is accorded considerable priority in social work ethics because clients have a lot to lose, a lot to risk, and a lot to be deprived of through their relationships to social workers, not the least of which is the service they happen to need. Impaired capacity to provide such service because of inebriation or addiction is but one of the problems social work ethics provide for.

Because of their condition, their need, their problems, and their circumstances, clients are susceptible to exploitation—financially, sexually, and in other ways. Often, they do not have to be totally defenseless to become victims of the power or influence of social workers who choose to abuse it.

Social work ethics provide for affirmative expectations as well as restraints and prohibitions. Availing clients of service and affording them access to it, without bias, discrimination, or prejudice, is a basic expectation of social workers. They are also expected to respect the confidences, the privacy, and the autonomy of clients.

To safeguard the rights of clients, social workers are importuned to avoid conflicting interests and loyalties that might prevent them from unequivocally devoting their efforts and attention to clients. They are also advised to avoid developing vested interests in outcomes for clients to such an extent that their own professional judgment becomes impaired or the preferences of clients are neglected.

Fairness in setting fees, without extraneous influences like paying others for referral or splitting fees, is an additional admonition in social work ethics. Provision is made for the consideration of clients' ability to pay, and appropriate referral if necessary to suit their circumstances.

If social workers find it necessary to violate these or other provisions of social work ethics, they must be prepared with a rationale convincing enough to demonstrate that the violation was indeed urgent in light of conflicting priorities or superseding values. These are better identified as considerations before the fact rather than retroactive justifications.

Social Workers and Their Colleagues

Whatever their formal assignments and tasks in organizational or interorganizational structures of one kind or another, or even in their own practice as private practitioners, social workers relate to others as associates or colleagues. As participants in intraorganizational or interorganizational staff groups, shared offices, professional associations, or self-help professional groups, social workers incur, or have attributed to them, ethical responsibilities to one another. Their cooperation is expected, as is their commitment to collective ends.

They may differ about goals or means to their attainment, and they may even find themselves in conflict regarding their ethical responsibility to peers, associates, and employers, but they are expected to avoid undermining the efforts and standing or credibility of peers and associates, however informal and extracurricular their relationships or associations. This does not preclude the necessity which may arise to intervene responsibly to prevent peers or associates from engaging in unethical conduct, or to participate in disciplinary proceedings when others are alleged to have done so.

In their work and relationships with colleagues, both in their own settings and in others, social workers are expected to be fair, civil, and cooperative. Confidences shared by colleagues are re pected, and their achievements and qualifications accurately reported. Complaints and criticisms of colleagues—including those about their ethics—must be responsibly lodged. Channels must be used that have been established and designed for them, with care taken for their substantiation, and with attention to fairness and due process.

As supervisors and superiors of colleagues, social workers are expected to facilitate their efforts and their professional development. They are to render fair and accurate judgments and evaluations of others' work.

Social workers who are colleagues in an organization or an endeavor have access to information about one another that they would not otherwise have. Some of it is private and confidential. Particular discretion and restraint are required regarding where and how such information is used and toward what end, not to mention *whether* the information is used at all.

Awareness of a colleague's life style (like one's sexual orientation or unconventional living arrangements) that results from professional association or sheer personal proximity, and that bears no relevance to professional responsibility and performance, is not properly communicated to others without that colleague's express approval. It is certainly not communicated with the intention or effect of contaminating that colleague's professional standing or effectiveness, and certainly not for the purpose of one's own personal or professional aggrandizement. What information is appropriate for administrative consideration in relation to the accredited goals of an agency or an enterprise is something for administrators and leaders of the agency or enterprise to discover, assuming ethical procedures and due process, and to use if relevance to professional performance can be demonstrated.

How colleagues deal with one another, relate to one another, and treat one another is a matter of particular ethical concern. Beyond the expectation of cooperation in the interest of achieving shared professional and organizational goals, is the ethical responsibility to avoid such behavior and relationships as may reflect or cast doubt on professional judgment and objectivity. A love affair or personal animosity between colleagues that colors their actions or evaluations, or intrudes on their capacity to work effectively and harmoniously together, is an ethical as well as administrative hazard.

Sexual overtures, sexual harassment, and other demeaning forms of disrespect and ridicule, even in informal circumstances, let alone work situations, are as ethically unacceptable among peers as they are in administrative and supervisory relationships.

In effect, the circumstances in which colleagues find themselves while performing their professional functions, and the effects they can have on one another to the detriment of their shared enterprise or to the detriment or discomfort of one another, dictate scrupulous and attentive regard to their ethics. This is true no matter how competent and proficient their professional functioning in their performance of their assigned tasks may otherwise be.

Social Workers and Their Employers

Social work ethics require social workers' loyalty to employers, and a conscientious effort to fulfill their responsibility to them. Included is adherence to employer policies and procedures (barring illegal, fraudulent, destructive, or discriminatory actions that might justify exceptions). While performing their assigned functions, social workers are expected to be guided by the purposes and goals of their employers. They are expected to use material, structural, financial, and personnel resources considerately and economically for the administrative and service purposes intended.

Social Workers and the Social Work Profession

As members of the social work profession, social workers share responsibility for the profession's reputation and standing in society, and its contributions to society; for its effective functioning as a service profession; and for the continued development of knowledge relevant to social work practice and education. Social workers share responsibility for representing and living up to the values of the profession, and for advancing the ethics to which it subscribes, by abiding by its code of ethics in their own professional conduct, and by encouraging and inducing others to do so.

Individual social workers, along with their colleagues and professional associations, are expected to contribute their own time, effort, and talents to the improvement of society and the lot of its poor, sick, disabled, deprived, and disadvantaged. As members of the social work profession they also share a commitment to eliminate discrimination in society. They strive to ensure access for all its constituents to resources, services, opportunities, entitlements, and options appropriate to their rights, needs, conditions, capacities, and circumstances.

This brief review of the substance of social work ethics hardly exhausts its subject matter as it may already be formulated in codes of social work ethics, or as it may have to be conjured in a moment of decision during the practice of social work. Considered along with the multifarious circumstances of practice, the diversity of participants in its processes, and the persons and interests affected by them, ethical judgments in any situation are, at least, a challenge. They require considerable thought, and contention with considerable uncertainty, with rarely the leisure that social workers might feel they need to do justice to the issues they face in many practice situations. The paradigm to be proposed for this purpose may do little to speed up the process, and perhaps less to increase the confidence of social workers in it. However, it should help suggest the issues and considerations they need to be aware of in order to be as thorough as they can in the time and circumstances at their disposal, and in order to make the best and most suitable ethical judgments they are capable of.

Chapter III

Making Ethical Judgments in Social Work Practice

Although ethical judgments in social work practice must often be made quickly and in the heat and turmoil of some practice situations, they must be made with sufficient thought and care to afford social workers a degree of assurance and conviction about their aptness and applicability. They must also be amenable to validation as appropriate and timely, preferably before the fact but also afterwards, should that be required by an adjudication of an unethical conduct complaint or other proceeding or inquiry.

The major criterion for evaluating a social worker's decisions and actions in a practice situation is that they be ethical in and for the circumstances in which they occur. They should also adequately and appropriately reflect the social worker's consideration of service goals and professional responsibilities.

Decisions and actions that are ethical may or may not be given precedence over those that are most consistent with service goals and professional responsibilities, but social work ethics require that both the ethics and the practice goals of a situation be considered and accounted for before conclusions are reached. A systematic rationale would be required to validate the choice of one over the other when provision for both is impossible in the situation.

COLLECTING AND WEIGHING THE FACTS

In any social work practice situation, awareness and consideration of all the relevant facts are essential for purposes of both competent and ethical professional performance, and for the effective exercise of professional discretion and judgment. Relevant facts include the functions and job descriptions of social workers, and the short- and long-range goals toward which they are working in relation to clients and others.

Awareness of specific data (like age), general circumstances of clients, and the impact of other persons and influences on clients, as well as the impact of clients and their actions on them, is also a prerequisite to ethical practice, just as it is for competent practice.

In contending with any practice situation social workers must be mindful of any biases, preferences or pressures that may skew their perspective of the facts, or selective attention to them.

Objectivity is essential, not disinterest or indifference, but the capacity to observe, interpret, and appraise the facts accurately and realistically. This is necessary in order to select those reactions and interventions that are ethically as well as practically most appropriate for, and applicable to, each situation, and to short- and long-range practice goals.

Facts relevant to ethics and to practice include the types of clients affected, their specific needs and conditions, their emotional and intellectual capacities, etc. — facts that help social workers determine the principles of ethics that apply to each situation, and whether and how they are to be applied. Principles of social work ethics, like principles of social work practice, may require tempering or modification even when their selection for application is indicated. Particular circumstances and personal capacities, along with other variables, must be taken into account before final decisions are made and actions taken by social workers.

IDENTIFYING LOCI AND LEVELS
OF ETHICAL RESPONSIBILITY

Sometimes the choice of principles of ethics to apply in a practice situation is neither clear nor self-evident. Social workers must therefore review the entire range of principles that may be applicable in any situation and the range of those to whom they may be applicable. Selections must then be made for maximum relevance and applicability, and priorities ordered among the applicable principles and those to whom they apply.

The choice between ethical actions and manifestly unethical ones poses few difficulties for social workers. Unless, of course, they are tempted or inclined toward unethical ones (for reasons of self-interest, for example). More difficult is the choice between actions regarded as equally ethical in relation to different persons or interests, equally considerate of different work assignments or goals, or equally compatible with different principles of ethics, and when the choices are mutually exclusive or cannot be concurrently accommodated.

The following case illustrates such a conflict of choices. A five-year-old child was formerly the client of a social worker who had sexually molested him. His parents refused to press charges of unethical conduct against the former social worker, or to permit the current social worker to do so. The age of the client makes it difficult, if not inappropriate, for the current social worker to leave the decision up to the client. On the other hand, the social worker's ethical responsibility as a member of the social work profession to intervene in a case of unethical conduct by a social worker does not give her leave to ignore or neglect the problem. Yet her accountability to the client's parents requires consideration of, and respect for, the parents' wishes and right to self-determination, if not in their own right, then in their capacity as the client's caretakers and guardians. Nevertheless, the values and interests of society compel the social worker to be concerned about the protection of defenseless and vulnerable minors. In this case, however, the alleged acts have already taken place, so that the issue is less the protection of the client than the disciplining of the former social worker and the prevention of further unethical conduct.

Since all of these possibilities imply conflicting responsibilities for the current social worker, her choices require the neglect of some of her options. The setting of priorities can therefore be an agonizing process; additionally, as is true of ethical judgments in most practice situations, not all social workers are likely to agree on one or another conclusion. It is incumbent upon each social worker, therefore, to pay scrupulous attention to all of the facts, issues, and applicable principles of ethics when arriving at ethical judgments and acting upon them. This conception of responsibility is consistent with that of Hobart:

As regards the origin of the term, a man is responsible when he is the person to respond to the question why the act was performed, how it is to be explained or justified. That is what he must answer, he is answerable for the act. It is the subject for which he must give an account; he is accountable for the act. The act proceeded from him. He is to say whether it proceeded consciously. He is to give evidence that he did or did not know the moral nature of the act, and that he did or did not intend the result. He is to say how he justifies it or if he can justify it.[1]

Within the context of the practice situation in which ethical judgments must be made, scrutiny of facts, issues, and principles is best done before the judgments are made and actions taken, and not await the need for subsequent justification. Also indicated is consideration of the probable consequences of the actions to be taken, and the professional skills that may be required to deal with them.

UTILITY OF PARADIGM IN MAKING ETHICAL JUDGMENTS

The pressure to make ethical judgments can indeed be overwhelming, not only for students and novices, but also for skilled and experienced social workers. Simply accounting for all the data relevant to practice situations, and to ethical judgments in them, is challenge enough, let alone making the best and the right choices with due regard for both social work ethics and social work goals. On the other hand, because of their work in society, the formal or informal sanctions accorded to perform it, and the risks and stakes attending it, social workers cannot escape making ethical judgments. They must do so in a rational manner comprehensible to others, including clients, peers, employers, professional associations, and so on. Plausible and practical standards and guidance are desirable to assist them in the process.

---

1. R. E. Hobart, "Free Will as Involving Determination and Inconceivable Without It." In Bernard Berofsky, ed., *Free Will and Determination* (New York: Harper and Row, 1966), pp. 90, 92.

Codes of social work ethics can be helpful, but they are rarely the final word, either in content or formulation. Professional discretion is still necessary in each practice situation. A paradigm to guide social workers through the process of making ethical judgments could do a great deal to increase the likelihood that all the pertinent factors of practice situations are given the attention and analysis they merit. Toward this end, the following paradigm is offered:

1. What principles of ethics are applicable in the practice situation, and to whom (or to what) are they applicable?
2. In relation to the social worker's primary responsibilities, how may priorities be justifiably ordered when ranking both the applicable principles of ethics and those (persons and interests) to whom they are applicable?
3. What are the risks and probable consequences to be taken into account by the social worker when making ethical judgments in a practice situation?
4. What considerations and values are sufficiently compelling to supersede the principles of ethics that might otherwise be suited to the practice situation?
5. What provisions and precautions will be required of the social worker in order to cope with the consequences of the social worker's ethical judgments and actions?
6. How can the contemplated decisions and actions be evaluated in the context of ethical and professional responsibility?

The objective for the social worker would be to pose these questions during confrontations with issues of ethics in practice situations. The social worker should contend with them as thoroughly, quickly, and exhaustively as necessary and possible for the purpose of reaching a maximally ethical conclusion.

By way of illustration and example, a series of vignettes will be presented in the next chapter to which this paradigm will be applied.

Chapter IV

Application of Paradigm
in Social Work Practice

The vignettes that follow are adapted from observations, experiences, news reports, and other sources. They will be used to demonstrate the application of the previously outlined paradigm to ethical judgments in social work practice. Since they are but glimpses of practice situations, the data available for scrutiny and consideration as a basis for arriving at ethical judgments is limited when compared with data normally available to social workers in complete records of a case or assignment. These illustrations are merely suggestive of the kind of thought and deliberation that might go into the ethical analysis of social work practice. They do not dwell on the other practice considerations that would also be necessary.

Obviously, these illustrations cannot exhaust the range of ethical issues that social workers are likely to encounter in their daily work, in the variety of roles they are called upon to perform, and in the variety of assignments and settings in which they are performed. They should therefore be examined with these realistic limitations in mind.

Analyses by different social workers of the incidents and situations presented, for their ethical import and implications, may differ in either the issues and principles viewed as pertinent and as meriting priority or in the evaluation of the ethical judgments made. The ultimate test of the validity of the choices made in actual experience would be whether they can indeed be substantiated and justified. They must make sense as premises for the actions of social workers and as a basis for appraisal by unbiased and impartial peers in the context of the specific practice situations.

Procedures are necessary and must be available to permit investigation and adjudication of complaints and grievances by fair, credible, and impartial groups with power and authority enough to deal with charges of unethical conduct. The effects sought would not only be to discipline and punish unethical conduct but also, by their actions and rulings, to illuminate the requisites of ethical conduct. A by-product of their procedures might also be increased trustworthiness of the social work profession. The Committees on Inquiry of the National Association of Social Workers and the Association's Board of Directors (which reviews the decisions of local committees on appeal) are such groups.

The illustrations should be used for purposes of discussion and deliberation, and as examples of the methods that may be employed in social work experience on the line.

SOCIAL WORKER'S PERSONAL COMPORTMENT

Mr. Wilson,* a social worker in private practice, attended a Thanksgiving Day party given in celebration of his forthcoming marriage. In the conviviality of the occasion, he drank more than he was accustomed to or could tolerate. Checking his answering machine, he heard a rather desperate message from Mrs. Colen. She was a client he had been seeing, on Thursdays, since the recent death of her husband to help her cope with her loss which had been devastating to her. Mr. Wilson had prepared her for the holiday cancellation but encouraged her to telephone him if she needed to. She insisted that she had to see him and urged him to return her call as soon as he possibly could to arrange the meeting.

Applicable Principles of Ethics

The social worker's primary responsibility is to his client. In communicating and meeting with his client, he has the ethical responsibility to be in full control of himself and his professional judgment. Moreover, he has the ethical responsibility to conduct himself, in his professional capacity and status, in a manner that

---

*All names used in these vignettes are fictitious.

does not reflect adversely upon himself as a social worker or upon the social work profession.

Priority of Applicable Principles

Mr. Wilson is expected to accord priority to Mrs. Colen's needs and interests, and to be in full possession of his emotional and intellectual faculties while attending to them.

Risks to be Taken into Account and Provided For

A major risk is the harm that might come to Mrs. Colen if her cry for help is neglected or dealt with inadequately. Mr. Wilson's venturing a prompt response to her call while under the influence of alcohol risks impaired and probably inappropriate communication. The possible consequence is damaged professional credibility and status both for Mr. Wilson as a social worker and for the social work profession as a whole. Under the circumstances, arranging to see her augments the risks for both Mrs. Colen and Mr. Wilson.

Superseding Values

No value would appear to supersede that of timely and effective response to Mrs. Colen's need for help, or of Mr. Wilson's responsibility to be in condition and to have the unimpaired capacity to provide it.

Provisions and Precautions

Although Mr. Wilson may be regarded as entitled to conduct himself as he pleases when he is not performing his professional role as a social worker, he is not ethically free to ignore Mrs. Colen's need for his help. On the other hand, talking to her on the telephone with slurred speech or other indications of impaired capacity might give Mrs. Colen reason to doubt his readiness to be helpful, and make her apprehensive about being under his care. Simply calling back must be carefully considered.

If Mr. Wilson has not already provided for coverage of his cases during his absence, he should try to provide for it. He should arrange for another social worker or other practitioner to call or see Mrs. Colen and to explain that Mr. Wilson was not in a position to call or see her immediately, but would contact her about an appointment as soon as possible. If another reliable and reputable social worker or other practitioner cannot be found, then Mr. Wilson should at least arrange for another reliable person to make the call. If one is found, a judgment can be made, from how Mrs. Colen sounds, about the urgency of seeing her promptly. It may be that she will be able to wait for Mr. Wilson's availability. A better course of action would be for Mr. Wilson, aware of the potential for such emergencies on holidays during which clients are apt to feel especially lonely and depressed, not to drink or otherwise indulge himself to the point that he is not equal to emergencies that may arise or that can be anticipated. And he should make reliable arrangements for emergencies when he is not accessible.

Evaluation

The important objective in this situation is to ensure the kind of intervention for Mrs. Colen that she needs when she needs it. If any suicidal inclination is even remotely detected — and here awareness and consideration of her history are crucial — then prompt and careful action is imperative.

TRUTH IN CREDENTIALS

Mr. Warren, a second-year student in a graduate school of social work, is placed for field instruction in the Montrose Mental Health Service under the supervision of Ms. Stone. Most of Montrose's clients are emotionally troubled. Mr. Warren expresses to Ms. Stone his concern about admitting to his assigned clients that he is a student, for fear that they would not have enough confidence in him to make his practice effective.

Applicable Principles of Ethics

Social workers are ethically responsible to be truthful about their professional status and credentials. Social work supervisors are ethically responsible to require ethical practice of supervisees, and to inspire and assist them in their development as ethical as well as competent social workers. Both are ethically responsible for competent and ethical service to clients.

Priority of Applicable Principles

Service to clients merits Mr. Warren's and Ms. Stone's highest ethical priority. In stating his qualifications, Mr. Warren neither lies about nor exaggerates his credentials. Nor does he imply that they are other than they actually are. Neither does Ms. Stone mislead Mr. Warren's clients about them.

Ms. Stone also has the ethical responsibility to ensure learning experiences and opportunities for Mr. Warren that are conducive to his becoming both ethical and competent, while providing safeguards for the protection of Mr. Warren's clients and service to them.

Risks to be Taken into Account and Provided For

There are risks for Mr. Warren's clients since Mr. Warren is still a student and presumably less than fully qualified. There are also risks for the reputation of the Montrose Mental Health Service and Ms. Stone as a consequence of inadequate performance by Mr. Warren or dishonesty on his part while he is learning to be a social worker and developing his skills.

Superseding Values

There is no question about the priority of ethical responsibility owed by the Montrose Mental Health Service, Ms. Stone, and Mr. Warren to clients. However, though perhaps not a value that clearly supersedes their ethical responsibility to clients, the value of providing learning opportunities for social work students is an important one. This is especially true in view of the need to prepare future generations of social workers for competent and ethical service to future generations of clients.

Provisions and Precautions

Mr. Warren's concern about acknowledging his status as a student can serve as a basis for discussing his ethical responsibility to be truthful when stating his professional credentials. Ms. Stone can provide Mr. Warren with the guidance and support he may need to help him deal with clients' reactions and concerns about not being treated by a fully qualified social worker. Ms. Stone should also reassure clients, directly or through Mr. Warren, or both, that safeguards would be in place at all times and that, in addition, Mr. Warren would always have access to Ms. Stone and to other supports as well as the resources of collateral educational experience.

Evaluation

In dwelling on the ethical implications of these and other issues, Ms. Stone sensitizes Mr. Warren to the ethics of social work practice and becomes, in effect, teacher and role model for Mr. Warren. Implicit in these processes is the emphasis for Mr. Warren on the great responsibility he carries in relation to clients, and the cautions it requires for client protection, and provision of adequate and ethical service.

INCAPACITATED SUPERVISEE

Mr. Wallace is a clinical social worker in the Alcott Social Agency, which serves persons with drug problems. He is supervised by Ms. Simon. Ms. Simon has heard rumors that Mr. Wallace uses controlled substances but has not seen evidence of his doing so either in or outside of the agency. She has also seen no evidence of his impairment because of drug use.

Applicable Principles of Ethics

Social workers are ethically responsible not to engage in social work practice while under the influence of alcohol or controlled substances, or when professional judgment and competence are impaired. Their personal conduct outside of their professional role and status is their own business unless and until such conduct compromises or otherwise interferes with the fulfillment of their professional responsibilities to clients, agency, and the social work profession. Supervisors of social workers have the ethical responsibility to safeguard the well-being of their supervisees' clients, and to ensure competent performance of assigned professional functions.

Priority of Applicable Principles

Mr. Wallace's and Ms. Simon's primary responsibility is to Mr. Wallace's clients. Mr. Wallace and Ms. Simon also have the ethical responsibility to perform their assigned professional functions, and to adhere to the Alcott Social Agency's policies and procedures. In addition, Ms. Simon is ethically accountable for monitoring and facilitating Mr. Wallace's performance at the Alcott Social Agency.

Risks to be Taken into Account and Provided For

The Alcott Social Agency's clients are at risk in relation to problems and vulnerabilities associated with addictive drugs. Mr. Wallace's privacy and professional reputation, and perhaps his opportunity to practice social work, are also at risk without just cause, should the rumor that he indulges in drugs prove to be false. If there is any foundation to the rumor, there is the risk of the impaired performance of his agency functions, with potentially harmful consequences for his clients and for the Alcott Social Agency.

Superseding Values

The right of privacy, including Mr. Wallace's right to privacy, is an exalted value in American society, but one not sufficiently exalted to be accorded precedence over the well-being of Mr. Wallace's clients and his appropriate and competent treatment of them. Neither does it merit priority over the credibility of the social work profession and of the Alcott Social Agency as media for the treatment of drug problems.

Provisions and Precautions

Ms. Simon should not rely on rumors or other insufficiently reliable sources of information concerning Mr. Wallace's conduct and practice as they may affect his role in the Alcott Social Agency or in the social work profession. Under optimal circumstances, as a matter of pedagogical and developmental dynamics in social work supervision, the supervisee is usually the primary source of information for the supervisor about the supervisee's own practice. However, it may be supplemented by observation and other normal agency opportunities. The supervisor then makes the most constructive use possible of the information in order to evaluate and assist in the improvement of the supervisee's performance and service to clients.

In this situation, however, while Ms. Simon may not be relying on rumor, she must be alert to signs of impaired performance and to signs of external intrusion on Mr. Wallace's capacity to meet professional and agency requirements, not so much to make judgments about what causes problems in performance, but about the possibility that such problems exist.

On the other hand, since Mr. Wallace is working with clients with histories of drug problems, extraordinary caution is required on Ms. Simon's part. Prompt attention must be paid to any manifestation of problems that pose specific hazards for clients, and their prospects for recovery, because these problems may affect clients and their needs. Questions must at least be raised about a social worker with a possible drug problem who is assigned to help clients with drug problems. Perhaps Ms. Simon should directly question Mr. Wallace, especially if there is any indication that there may be such a problem.

If there is evidence of impaired performance, Ms. Simon's intervention would be essential, if not to prevent Mr. Wallace from practicing, because of the seriousness of the problem, then to put Mr. Wallace on notice that the level of practice that is evident is not acceptable and, whatever the cause, Mr. Wallace must attend to it immediately. However, if in addition, the rumor about Mr. Wallace's indulging in drugs is confirmed, Ms. Simon would have to insist with an offer of help, that Mr. Wallace go for treatment. Perhaps this would take the form of paid temporary leave, with provision for the resumption of Mr. Wallace's duties upon successful completion of treatment.

Evaluation

Mr. Wallace's clients are the primary concern for Ms. Simon, but Mr. Wallace also merits Ms. Simon's concern and assistance, both in his own right and in his role as a social worker, as long as it is not at the expense of clients or with risk to them and the treatment for which they resort to the Alcott Social Agency. Intervention which takes both into account, along with the interests of the Alcott Agency and the community, would appear to be both judicious and considerate.

SOCIAL WORKER'S PUBLIC IMAGE

Ms. Warner, a social worker employed by the Adams Social Service Agency, has published a book on parent-child relations which has received considerable public attention. She is asked by a local radio station to conduct a regularly scheduled program during which listeners would be invited to ask for her advice about their problems. Her introduction would include her agency affiliation.

Applicable Principles of Ethics

Social workers are ethically responsible to keep their public conduct and statements in their capacity and status as members of the social work profession above reproach. They are also expected to distinguish between their actions and statements as private citizens and those as agency representatives. They are ethically responsible as well for the exercise of care and caution in the kind and substance of their public actions and statements.

Priority of Applicable Principles

A primary ethical concern for Ms. Warner is the effect of her actions and statements in her role and status as a social worker on others, including the effect on the Adams Social Service Agency and on the image of the social work profession.

Risks to be Taken into Account and Provided For

Listeners might assume Ms. Warner is speaking for the Adams Social Service Agency. Her responses to listeners' questions about their problems in family relationships may be taken literally and acted on, even if they are not intended to be. Since the responses are based on necessarily limited and possibly skewed data, without benefit of a carefully and purposefully developed professional relationship, they are subject to the risk of faulty diagnosis and planning. The result may be a simplistic and inaccurate perception of social work.

Superseding Values

Whatever the possibility of public relations value for Ms. Warner, the Adams Social Service Agency, and the social work profession in the proposed broadcasts, it should not be accorded precedence over either the potential harm to listeners or the integrity of social work as an approach to meeting human need.

Provisions and Precautions

Whether Ms. Warner undertakes the broadcasts, and regardless of what she says on them if she does, she must take into account the risks that inhere in them and act accordingly. She must certainly not permit herself to be unduly tempted by the prospect of personal fame and rewards in deciding whether to do the broadcasts. If she does decide to do them, in the introduction and publicity for them, she should provide for the controls and limits necessary to avoid risks and misunderstandings for listeners or inappropriate and hazardous actions by them. The fact that she is not representing or speaking for the Adams Social Service Agency or the social work profession must be underscored.

Evaluation

The proposed precautions are essential to avoid consequences that may be dysfunctional for the Adams Social Service Agency and the social work profession, both of which have a considerable stake in Ms. Warner's public actions and statements.

SOCIAL WORKER'S PERSONAL SAFETY

Seven-year-old Tommy is in the temporary care of a protective service, pending resolution of the custody battle between his parents. Ms. Whelan is the social worker assigned to Tommy. From what Tommy has intimated, not without difficulty, and from what she has observed in her contacts with him, she has become aware of his father's repeated abuse of him.

Shortly before the adjudication of the custody case, Tommy's father (a man with obvious violent tendencies) accosts Ms. Whelan and threatens to kill her, her husband, and her two small children, if her testimony prevents him from obtaining custody of Tommy. Tommy has agreed that her truthful testimony is important to his well-being, and encouraged her to provide it.

Applicable Principles of Ethics

The social worker's primary ethical responsibility is to her client. She is also ethically responsible for telling the truth in testimony that affects her endangered minor client and his future care. This is true only if she has been given or, according to the definition of her professional function, is assumed to have permission to testify as to her work with the client and her knowledge of his circumstances.

Priority of Applicable Principles

Tommy's safety and well-being are of primary professional and ethical concern for Ms. Whelan. As a wife and parent, she does have a concern and responsibility for the safety of herself and her family, but not to the extent of justifying neglect of her responsibility to Tommy. She is also ethically responsible for conscientious and unbiased performance of her assigned role during the custody proceeding and toward the goal of a result in Tommy's best interests.

Risks to Be Taken into Account and Provided For

One of the issues affecting Ms. Whelan's ethical responsibility as a social worker is the possibility that custody may be awarded to Tommy's father with the probability of future abuse. There is also the risk of unjust consequences from her testimony if it is not truthful or accurate. The risk for Ms. Whelan and her family is also a real one.

Superseding Values

The guiding value for Ms. Whelan is that associated with ethical responsibility to and for the safety and well-being of Tommy, a child as well as a client. Although meriting concern and provision, the threat to the lives of Ms. Whelan and her family would not, as a matter of social work ethics, be accorded superseding priority.

Provisions and Precautions

Ms. Whelan is ethically responsible for the competent performance of her professional role in relation to her client, Tommy, whose age and vulnerability require every precaution regarding his protection and well-being. Her role in the custody proceeding is to provide such relevant evidence as she can confidently and accurately offer, with the particular caution that the best interests of Tommy must be adequately provided for. As for the threat to herself and her family, she should resort to the authorities and any other resource for intervention and protection. She should also exercise every other precaution necessary to protect herself and her family.

Evaluation

In spite of the apparent injustice to Ms. Whelan and her family in these measures, they are compelled by Ms. Whelan's prior professional responsibility to Tommy, given the prospective effect of her testimony on his best interests. Social workers do relinquish much of their autonomy and self-interest because of their commitment to their professional and ethical social work responsibility.

LIMITS ON CONFIDENTIALITY

Ms. Worley is a social caseworker at the Argon Family Service Agency. After a rather general screening by an intake worker, Ms. Carroll is assigned to Ms. Worley for treatment. In their first session, Ms. Carroll expresses concern about the possible revelation of her confidences, and seeks from Ms. Worley assurance that under no circumstances will Ms. Worley share them with anyone else. Ms. Worley, however, is required by the agency to keep records of her work with Ms. Carroll and to discuss them with her supervisor.

Applicable Principles of Ethics

The principle of confidentiality applies to the relationship between social worker and client. The social worker is also ethically responsible to tell the client the truth about those agency policies and procedures that will limit the extent to which she will be free to honor the principle of confidentiality. In addition, the social worker is ethically responsible to be clear and forthright about the manner in which treatment will be conducted, and the roles that both social worker and client will be playing. The social worker respects the client's right to self-determination in all matters affecting the client's life.

Priority of Applicable Principles

The principle of confidentiality merits Ms. Worley's priority. Also pertinent are Ms. Worley's respect for Ms. Carroll's right to self-determination and Ms. Worley's truthfulness with regard to agency policies and procedures (and Ms. Worley's practices) that may affect Ms. Carroll's experience and opportunities as her client.

Risks to Be Taken into Account and Provided For

Failure by Ms. Worley to candidly share information with Ms. Carroll regarding the circumstances under which she and Ms. Carroll will be operating risks undermining her trust in Ms. Worley and evoking her doubts about Ms. Worley and the Argon Family Service Agency's credibility. If Ms. Worley does not withhold any of the relevant information, Ms. Carroll may decide that the policies and procedures outlined do not accord with her needs and preferences. She may then refuse to receive treatment from the agency, although she may need it desperately. There is inevitably the risk of carelessness or misuse of records and other information, especially, but not exclusively, in a large agency.

Superseding Values

Ms. Carroll's need for treatment, which Ms. Worley's values as a social worker cause her to be concerned about, would not be a sufficient reason for Ms. Worley to compromise her ethical responsibility to be truthful about the circumstances of Ms. Carroll's treatment, should she proceed with it.

Provisions and Precautions

Ms. Worley truthfully anticipates with Ms. Carroll the kinds of experiences and demands she can expect as her client and as a client of the Argon Family Service Agency. She does so in a business-like fashion not to avoid intimidation, but rather to make clear their connection to the purposes of treatment. Ms. Worley's recordings and discussions with her supervisor can be described as resources and controls that are designed to be used in Ms. Carroll's interests, and are neither arbitrary nor intended to be used for any other purposes. She may have to acknowledge that accidents do happen but that precautions are taken to avoid them. Ms. Worley emphasizes that information from and about Ms. Carroll is shared only with those who have legitimate business with it, and that she intends to keep it confidential as far as anybody else is concerned. At the same time, she admits that that information is not her exclusive property since, as an agency employee, she is under the agency's administrative constraints. She adds that whether Ms. Carroll subjects herself to the conditions outlined is something for her to decide. They do deserve her careful consideration. If a practical and satisfactory alternative is available for Ms. Carroll to choose, referral is appropriate.

Evaluation

As important as it is, the principle of confidentiality is rarely absolute, and certainly not in social work practice within agencies and institutions. Ms. Carroll is entitled to know the risks to it as well as anything else she might need to know in order to make an intelligent and well-considered judgment about whether or not to receive Ms. Worley's and the agency's services.

COLLUSION BETWEEN SOCIAL WORKER AND CLIENT

Mr. Crane admits to Ms. Weller, his social worker in the Palm Public Assistance Agency, that he has been misleading the agency about his and his family's eligibility for financial and medical assistance. He asks Ms. Weller for the kind of cooperation he has received from other agency social workers so that aid is not terminated. He emphasizes that, as she must know, even with the aid he and his family are just on the edge of subsistence.

Applicable Principles of Ethics

The ethical principle of confidentiality applies to the relationship between social worker and client. The social worker is also ethically responsible to adhere to the purposes, policies and procedures of the agency which employs her.

Priority of Applicable Principles

Confidentiality remains a first principle of social work ethics for Ms. Weller, certainly with respect to information volunteered by Mr. Crane. On the other hand, Ms. Weller is ethically bound to not collaborate or connive with Mr. Crane in his fraudulent practices.

This applies to both the contravention of the Palm Agency's policies and procedures and the illegal and unethical resort to resources legislatively allotted for meeting human needs on an impartial and equitable basis.

Risks to Be Taken into Account and Provided For

Inherent in this situation is the risk of fraud in Mr. Crane's application for and receipt of the Palm Public Assistance Agency's financial and medical assistance. Ms. Weller may also be tempted to identify with Mr. Crane and to sympathize enough with him to cause her to bend or compromise the rules by which both she and Mr. Crane are bound. She may regard them as bureaucratic and unrealistic impediments to meeting genuine human needs.

Superseding Values

The value of providing for the actual needs of families in economic distress like Mr. Crane's can be a pressing one for Ms. Weller, as it might very well be for any social worker committed to social work ideology. However, Ms. Weller's ethical responsibilities to the Palm Public Assistance Agency, the community, and persons other than Mr. Crane and his family who are dependent on its resources, prevent Ms. Weller from putting relatively higher priority on that value as it applies to Mr. Crane.

Provisions and Precautions

Ms. Weller might have avoided contending with the issue of confidentiality by promptly informing Mr. Crane, upon the initiation of their relationship, that the Palm Agency's administrative regulations set precise limits on the application of the principle of confidentiality, for both Ms. Weller and Mr. Crane must abide by the agency's eligibility and procedural requirements. This can be done skillfully, and in a spirit of honesty and candor, rather than in a spirit of warning that might itself come through as a collusive hint. Sympathetic understanding can be expressed regarding the difficulty of meeting economic ends under existing welfare arrangements, with appreciation, at the same time, that equitable distribution must be made of the available funds. (Ms. Weller can engage in collective action with other social workers and various action groups to make more funds available and to influence the enactment of policies tailored to meet existing needs of the kind reflected in Mr. Crane's experience. She can also encourage Mr. Crane to do what he can toward the same end.)

The principle of confidentiality prevents Ms. Weller from simply communicating Mr. Crane's confidences, or using them to terminate the assistance Mr. Crane has been receiving. However, Ms. Weller can make clear to Mr. Crane that he cannot expect her to help him maintain the assistance or avert punitive action if data otherwise made available to the agency indicate that Mr. Crane is not eligible for the level of assistance he has been receiving. Ms. Weller would have the duty to encourage Mr. Crane to be accurate in his application for assistance.

Evaluation

The choices for Ms. Weller are limited, but her refusal to collaborate with the fraud or misstatements of Mr. Crane is an ethical response to the duty she owes to the Palm Public Assistance Agency without penalizing Mr. Crane for his own revelations, however misguided they might appear to be for his purposes. Mr. Crane would still be subject to agency regulations if his failure to meet eligibility requirements is subsequently admitted and verified. Ms. Weller would have the ethical responsibility to prepare him for this outcome.

CLIENT'S TELLING SOCIAL WORKER OF CRIME COMMITTED

In a session with his social worker, Mr. Walcott, Mr. Carne blurts out that he was the hit-and-run driver about whom Mr. Walcott had read in the newspaper. His car had seriously injured a teenage pedestrian, and he was drunk at the time. His purpose, he admitted, was less in expiation for the crime or out of concern about the fate of the pedestrian, than to solicit Mr. Walcott's help with his troubled conscience.

Applicable Principles of Ethics

The principle of confidentiality applies in this situation as does that of primacy of client's interests. The social worker also shares ethical concern about the effective administration of justice in the community.

Priority of Applicable Principles

Mr. Walcott's priority is normally given to the ethical responsibility to preserve Mr. Carne's volunteered confidences. He is also expected to accord primacy to Mr. Carne's interests. The effective administration of justice also merits some of his attention.

Risks to Be Taken into Account and Provided For

One risk that Mr. Carne would be concerned about is Mr. Walcott's revelation of his secret without his approval and with unwelcome consequences for him. Upon the injured pedestrian is imposed the risk of the pain, suffering, and deprivation that results from the accident, without possibility of recompense and restitution. For society, there is the risk of injustice from Mr. Carne's evasion of trial and punishment.

Superseding Values

As a social worker committed to the ideology of the social work profession, Mr. Walcott values justice and equity for persons criminally injured by individuals who have endangered the lives of others as well as themselves by driving while intoxicated. But confiding in Mr. Walcott, as Mr. Carne would be encouraged to do for the purpose of treatment according to the principle of confidentiality, raises questions about the validity of giving those values priority over Mr. Walcott's ethical responsibility to Mr. Carne.

Provisions and Precautions

Since the alleged crime to which Mr. Carne has confidentially confessed has already been committed — as contrasted with a serious crime one intends to commit with potential danger to others — Mr. Walcott cannot ethically justify the betrayal of Mr. Carne's confidences. Of course, he can and should use his professional skill to identify considerations that might influence Mr. Carne to consult a lawyer and perhaps take steps toward meeting his social responsibility to the injured pedestrian. As a reflection of his concern for Mr. Carne's own well-being, Mr. Walcott might suggest that Mr. Carne consider getting help for what appears to be a drinking problem.

Evaluation

Mr. Walcott's primary ethical responsibility is to Mr. Carne. He cannot, ethically, penalize Mr. Carne for admitting to his crime only because of the happenstance of his professional relationship to Mr. Walcott. On the other hand, for Mr. Walcott to neglect his concern about Mr. Carne's crime (and its potential repetition if he indeed has a drinking problem) or his concern about Mr. Carne's social values which prevent him from assuming responsibility for his actions, is to evade his responsibility as a social worker to society and its system of justice. He would at least be providing for these by confronting Mr. Carne without perpetrating a kind of blackmail made possible only because of their professional relationship.

MINOR CLIENT'S SECRETS

Fifteen-year-old Marty began a series of sessions with social worker Ms. Windom. His parents had suggested and agreed to pay for the sessions when they perceived an unhealthy tendency on his part to sulk and withdraw from social and family contacts. In an early session with Ms. Windom, Marty admitted his intention to "end it all." Ms. Windom took the admission seriously and urged Marty to consider voluntary hospitalization for psychiatric care.

When he refused, Ms. Windom told him that she would have to talk to his parents. Marty objected.

Applicable Principles of Ethics

The social worker has the ethical responsibility to respect the confidences and the right to self-determination of clients. The social worker owes clients primacy of their interests.

Priority of Applicable Principles

Marty's interests merit highest priority, but confidentiality and Marty's right to self-determination are principles of ethics to which Ms. Windom is also committed.

Risks to Be Taken into Account and Provided For

A major risk is to Marty's life, for he may indeed commit suicide as he threatens. In addition, a charge of malpractice or unethical conduct might be lodged against Ms. Windom by Marty's parents for failure to inform them of Marty's intention if they learn that Ms. Windom was aware of it, whether or not Marty actually does commit suicide. The betrayal of Marty's confidence, if Ms. Windom does inform them of Marty's intention, is likely to damage the treatment relationship between Marty and Ms. Windom, perhaps irreparably.

Superseding Values

The valuation of Marty's life is sufficiently compelling to require Ms. Windom to neglect her ethical commitment to the principle of confidentiality and respect for Marty's self-determination.

Provisions and Precautions

The risk to Marty's life necessitates Ms. Windom's consideration of unusual measures, including doing whatever she can to prevent his suicide and violating the principles of confidentiality and self-determination. If the prospect of the threatened suicide appears at all imminent, Ms. Windom would have to take the precipitous step of communicating with Marty's parents over Marty's objections so that they can consider involuntary commitment and anything else to ensure skilled and timely intervention for Marty.

Ms. Windom should do none of these things without stretching, to its practical outer limits, her opportunity to honor the principles of confidentiality and self-determination. However, the urgency of the crisis, her estimate of what constitutes the primacy of Marty's interests, and the fact that Marty is a minor whose capacity to exercise the judgment necessary to safeguard his own life may be in doubt, require that Ms. Windom compromise the principles of ethics to which she might otherwise give priority. Before doing so, she should respectfully engage Marty in a discussion of the reasons for her breach of confidentiality and its necessity as a matter of her professional responsibility.

Evaluation

The principal justifications for laying aside the principles of ethics that would normally be assigned priority are Marty's youthfulness and the circumstantial priority assigned to Marty's life which seems to be in real danger. There is the chance that Ms. Windom is mistaken about the imminence of the threat, but the valuation of Marty's life requires Ms. Windom to risk the possibility of error. Ms. Windom would then be deciding to err on the side of caution. The fact that Marty's parents have been paying the fees for Marty's treatment is not a justification for the course of action that Ms. Windom would be taking since it is nevertheless Marty who is Ms. Windom's client and not Marty's parents.

SUING CLIENT FOR NONPAYMENT OF FEES

Mr. Waring, a social worker, has been treating Mr. Cobb for several months. Since Mr. Cobb has shown considerable progress in coping with the problems that prompted him to seek help, Mr. Waring has recommended discontinuing treatment, and Mr. Cobb has agreed, with the understanding that he should feel free to call Mr. Waring if he needs to.

Mr. Cobb has ignored statements for, and reminders about, unpaid fees. When Mr. Waring has spoken to him, Mr. Cobb has insisted that he will not pay them. "Sue me," he has challenged.

Applicable Principles of Ethics

The social worker is normally committed to keeping confidential not only the difficulties for which the client is in treatment, but also the very fact that he is in treatment. The social worker also exercises restraint in resorting to legal procedures against the client for nonpayment so that confidentiality may be preserved.

Priority of Applicable Principles

Mr. Waring owes priority to the principle of confidentiality. However, Mr. Cobb has the reciprocal responsibility to cooperate with Mr. Waring to the maximum extent possible, with respect to both his participation in facilitating treatment and the payment of fees.

Risks to Be Taken into Account and Provided For

Suing Mr. Cobb for the unpaid fees risks revelation by Mr. Waring of Mr. Cobb's confidences as well as the fact that he has been in treatment with Mr. Waring. But his failure to pay the fees is at least an abrogation of Mr. Cobb's agreement to pay Mr. Waring for treatment. It may also be antithetical to Mr. Waring's treatment objectives if Mr. Cobb's difficulties have anything to do with a tendency toward irresponsibility.

Superseding Values

The value of fairness and justice for Mr. Waring in his claim to compensation for professional work done and time spent in treating Mr. Cobb does not exceed in importance the principle of confidentiality in social work ethics. Even in an involuntary appearance in a legal proceeding Mr. Waring has the ethical responsibility to resist pressure to violate it, let alone in a proceeding which he initiates for his own purposes. But it does merit some consideration.

Provisions and Precautions

The problem for Mr. Waring is to get the compensation to which he is entitled, and on which he relies for his sustenance, without violating the principle of confidentiality. Mr. Waring should therefore use a legal proceeding only as a last resort, giving Mr. Cobb as much opportunity as possible to make it unnecessary. If Mr. Waring does resort to legal action, he should share with the court (if required to advance the proceeding) only as much information as would be necessary to confirm the fact that Mr. Cobb was indeed in treatment with Mr. Waring for the period for which Mr. Waring seeks compensation. However, he should not reveal the substance of what transpired between them.

Evaluation

The solution to Mr. Waring's dilemma straddles the thin line between adhering to the principle of confidentiality and holding Mr. Cobb to the quid pro quo of the treatment arrangement.

Mr. Cobb has the right to waive the protection of the principle of confidentiality, and to grant or not to grant to Mr. Waring permission to reveal confidences shared by Mr. Cobb in their treatment sessions. By the same token, Mr. Cobb may be viewed as sharing responsibility with Mr. Waring for keeping them confidential. Just as Mr. Waring is not ethically free to use the principle of confidentiality — intended as a safeguard for the protection of Mr. Cobb and not Mr. Waring — to serve his own personal purposes rather than those of Mr. Cobb, Mr. Cobb should be limited in how he uses the principle to evade the responsibility of paying for services rendered. Other remedies are available to Mr. Cobb. if he can justify a claim of fraud, malpractice, or other deviation.

SOCIAL WORKER'S SOURCE
OF INFORMATION ABOUT CLIENT

Ms. Carver is a playwright who anticipates the opening of her new play. Ms. Winter, her social worker, would be interested in seeing Ms. Carver's play as a source of information about her that might be useful in treatment. The substance of the play, she thinks, might reveal material relevant to the process. The context of Ms. Carver's experience as a playwright, as Ms. Winter might be in a position to observe it, might afford her additional insight into Ms. Carver's needs and strengths. However, Ms. Carver has neither invited Ms. Winter to see the play nor suggested that she do so, in spite of Ms. Winter's expression of interest in it and enthusiasm about its production.

Applicable Principles of Ethics

In addition to the strategic utility of information about clients in planning clients' treatment, the social worker is ethically responsible to acquire and make use of such data as would enhance the social work treatment process. The social worker is also ethically responsible, as a matter of client self-determination, to be guided by clients' readiness and preferences regarding access to data about them.

Priority of Applicable Principles

Whatever the utility of seeing the play, for Ms. Winter and for the process of treating Ms. Carver, and despite Ms. Winter's ethical responsibility to acquire and use whatever information she may be able to get, Ms. Carver's right to self-determination regarding whether and how Ms. Winter gets the information is accorded priority when there is any reason for Ms. Winter to believe that Ms. Carver has any preference.

Risks to be Taken into Account and Provided For

Ms. Carver may indeed be reluctant to have Ms. Winter see the play for reasons that, if Ms. Winter can estimate them and if they can arise in their sessions together, could be dealt with therapeutically. However, if Ms. Winter does see the play, even with Ms. Carver's encouragement or invitation, there is a risk that Ms. Winter's response (perhaps upon Ms. Carver's urging) could detour or confuse the treatment purposes of their encounters. The play may be a poor one, for example, or Ms. Winter may not be able to hide her critical reaction to it. Silence itself might impress Ms. Carver as incriminating.

Superseding Values

Nothing is presented in the situation to indicate cause for violating the principles of ethics applicable to it; only the need to decide which of the principles to apply and how.

Provisions and Precautions

Playwrights, like other artists, tend to be sensitive about their creations. Ms. Winter must be cautious about the way in which she expresses interest in the forthcoming production, but she can hardly — at least justifiably — show no interest at all. Ms. Carver may have reasons to not want Ms. Winter to see the play, but she is not likely to take Ms. Winter's ignoring the prospect altogether with equanimity. Ms. Winter might find an uncharged moment to tactfully ask Ms. Carver if she would like her to see it. She could take into account the risks mentioned but prepare Ms. Carver for them. They can agree on how to handle the experience and how to employ it in their work together. One thing Ms. Winter should avoid if she does see the play is to transform herself into a drama critic. The data that might conceivably emerge for Ms. Winter upon seeing the play, if she did, are better revealed in her sessions with Ms. Carver and on Ms. Carver's terms, for use appropriate to their purposes together. A better opportunity to see that play or another one might come later as their purposes are achieved.

Evaluation

The needs and problems that have directed Ms. Carver to Ms. Winter, and Ms. Winter's professional function in relation to them, are central to Ms. Winter's professional relationship with Ms. Carver. Whether Ms. Carver's participation and responses in that relationship guide and determine Ms. Winter's performance of her role. Whether Ms. Carver's experience, prospects, and aspirations as a playwright properly become part of the substance of her interaction with Ms. Winter are options for Ms. Carver to exercise, although Ms. Winter provides avenues and opportunities for exploring them as Ms. Carver becomes ready for them.

REFERRING A CLIENT

Ms. Clark sought social worker Mr. Wynn's help with what she acknowledged to be a demeaning self-image, one which led her into very damaging relationships. Although she made some progress over a series of sessions in that she developed an increased capacity to cope constructively with her inclinations and even an increased self-acceptance, she revealed to Mr. Wynn a history of eating disorders that would subject her to relapses in her relationships and self-esteem. Because there was no clear evidence of a durable abatement of the disorder, and not feeling competent to treat it, Mr. Wynn considers a referral to someone who can.

Applicable Principles of Ethics

The social worker has the ethical responsibility to not undertake treatment of a client's problem for which the worker lacks the necessary competence. The social worker also has the ethical responsibility to neither terminate a treatment relationship prematurely nor continue it beyond the client's need for it or the social worker's capacity to treat the client effectively.

Priority of Applicable Principles

Of prior importance in the sequence of Mr. Wynn's ethical responsibilities is the availing to Ms. Clark of the mode of service most necessary and appropriate for her need, her quest, and her readiness, and in a manner maximally suited to her situation and her personal and material resources.

Risks to Be Taken into Account and Provided For

However appropriate referral may appear to be, because of Ms. Clark's need and because of Mr. Wynn's functional and professional limitations (assuming the necessary competence is available for her), referral may also represent rejection for Ms. Clark of a kind that she may have experienced and that may have caused her to suffer in the past. On the other hand, Mr. Wynn may be tempted to hang on to Ms. Clark as a client in a spirit of experimentation or maybe in response to a personal challenge, or perhaps because of ego or income needs.

Superseding Values

Mr. Wynn's ethical focus remains on the well-being of Ms. Clark, and the timely provision of competent service appropriate to her need and condition. No extraneous value supersedes that.

Provisions and Precautions

Though directing his attention to Ms. Clark emerging as well as existing needs, Mr. Wynn must proceed with caution. On one hand, he must not neglect a pressing need — as Ms. Clark evidently perceives it — namely, the eating disorder which makes her vulnerable to the difficulties that brought her to Mr. Wynn. On the other hand, he cannot disrupt the progress already made. That could be the result of Mr. Wynn's suggestion of referral. Mr. Wynn must also be clear and cautious about his own motivation when recommending referral or resisting it.

Evaluation

There does not seem to be any question about what needs to be done and what social work ethics require of Mr. Wynn. What Mr. Wynn must provide are timing, tact, and skill, along with self-awareness. The primacy of Ms. Clark's interests should not be neglected, nor should incidental harm accrue to her in providing for them.

CULTURE AS A VARIABLE
IN ETHICAL SOCIAL WORK PRACTICE

Mrs. Cross is a mother of six children who range in age from one to eight. She is disquieted and overwhelmed because she is pregnant again and dreads the physical and economic strain of an additional child. As a pious woman, she is conflicted about the option of abortion which is legally available and which she finds it hard to resist considering. As a member of a group which accords domestic authority to her husband, and knowing his and her group's aversion to abortion, she hesitates broaching the subject with him.

Hoping to find the rationale and courage to deal with her problem, which reality has compelled her to pursue, she applies to Ms. Winslow, a social worker, for help and counsel. Ms. Winslow is a pro-choice feminist with a personal zeal for the emancipation of women from household and child-rearing drudgery.

Applicable Principles of Ethics

The social worker is ethically responsible to perform her helping role with the client in a manner suited to the client's needs, wishes, and readiness, and compatible with her own professional function. Through her status as a social worker, she is also committed to the needs and rights of women in general.

Priority of Applicable Principles

Ms. Winslow owes priority to the needs and problems that Mrs. Cross presents to her, and with which she seeks social work assistance. Ms. Winslow also has the ethical responsibility to let Mrs. Cross's preferences guide her interventions.

Risks to Be Taken into Account and Provided For

Mrs. Cross's own ambivalence about an abortion and her fear of confronting her husband about one, or even suggesting it, may hamper her capacity to proceed with either course. Ms. Winslow's identification with Mrs. Cross's right to both, as well as her own personal investment in feminist causes, might incline her to encourage or urge Mrs. Cross to assert herself without readiness or conviction enough to do so. Upsetting consequences for Ms. Cross may result.

Superseding Values

Although feminist causes and opportunities for women represent high societal values for Ms. Winslow, and although these values are especially pertinent to Mrs. Cross, they are not predominant ones for Mrs. Cross. They are not predominant enough, at any rate, to preclude the operation of other values to which she subscribes.

Provisions and Precautions

Ms. Winslow has to guard against permitting her own zeal and commitments to induce Mrs. Cross to do what she lacks the will or conviction to do. The hazard is unanticipated and perhaps harmful consequences for which Mrs. Cross neither bargains nor is prepared. Ms. Winslow may help illuminate the options and alternatives available to Mrs. Cross but they, and their potential consequences, must be clearly delineated for Mrs. Cross's consideration and appraisal. This must be done before she makes what must be acknowledged to be her own freely made choices and for which she has complete responsibility.

Evaluation

By all available measures, the choice that Mrs. Cross ultimately makes may not be the best for her or even consistent with Ms. Winslow's carefully and objectively considered preferences for Mrs. Cross or for women in general. But, it is hers to make, whatever the consequences. If effects on others may be anticipated, then of course these, too, must be considered. Mrs. Cross does not give up her autonomy simply because she seeks social work help and counsel. Ms. Winslow can—and might even have the obligation to—do her work in the feminist cause in other settings.

INFLUENCES ON REFERRAL

Ms. Walsh is the senior social worker in Arlen Hospital, which includes in its patient load a high proportion of elderly and chronically ill persons. Arrow Nursing Home, a proprietary nursing home and one of the skilled nursing facilities to which Arlen Hospital's patients have been referred, has offered Ms. Walsh part-time employment as a social work consultant.

Applicable Principles of Ethics

Social workers have the ethical responsibility to base client referral on the needs and preferences of the clients (whether they act for themselves or delegate authority to others to act on their behalf) and on the appropriateness and applicability of the services to which they are referred. Concurrently serving two institutions that are parties to referral transactions is prima facie evidence of professionally unethical conduct.

Priority of Applicable Principles

The needs and preferences of Arlen Hospital patients scheduled for referral to skilled nursing facilities, and their right to self-determination in their choice of facilities, merit highest priority. This right applies to the extent that patients have the capacity to exercise it, or have had authority delegated to another to exercise it.

Ms. Walsh is ethically responsible for independent and unbiased judgment in suggesting needed services and facilities to patients (or if necessary, their representatives) and making them available for their consideration.

Risks to Be Taken into Account
and Provided For

In Ms. Walsh's selection and processing of patient referrals, her employment at Arrow Nursing Home creates the risk of appearing to be influenced by circumstances not maximally related to the needs and preferences of patients or their duly appointed surrogates. In addition, the potential bias toward Arrow Nursing Home, implicit in Ms. Walsh's employment there, would appear to disadvantage, without cause, other skilled nursing facilities. Access to these other facilities might very well be in the best interests of patients but, even if not, patients would be entitled to choose them if that is what they or their duly appointed surrogates wish.

Superseding Values

Independence of Ms. Walsh's professional judgment and its application in the service of patients (with due regard for right to self-determination and without the taint implicit in Ms. Walsh's serving two parties whose transactions affect patients) are values not contravened by other values.

Provisions and Precautions

Ms. Walsh should reject Arrow Nursing Home's offer of employment, with a clear statement of her reason, namely, that she would regard concurrent employment there as unethical. She should explain the risk to her credibility as a social worker and as an employee of Arlen Hospital. She might also want to assure the personnel at Arrow Nursing Home that the home would not be subject to reverse bias (arbitrary elimination as a potential referral resource as a consequence of the job offer, depending on her view of the implications of the job offer). Ms. Walsh's purpose behind spelling out her reasoning would be to reflect her ethical stance as a social worker, and as an employee of Arlen Hospital, in order to prevent the Arrow Nursing Home's personnel from perceiving her ethics as ambiguous or questionable.

Evaluation

The steps suggested would be consistent with those needed to both avoid the risks identified and, at the same time, emphasize — if only as a matter of education and orientation — some of the substance and rationale of social work ethics.

TRANSFER OF CLIENT

Ms. Cabel has been a client of Mr. Willet, a social worker in private practice for several months. Her progress with the difficulties that brought her to him has been quite evident. She informs him, with some hesitation, that she intends to switch to Ms. Worth, another social worker. She seems reluctant to spell out her reasons, but she is very clear about her desire to make the change, and she asks Mr. Willet to send Ms. Worth a summary of his work with her.

Mr. Willet has been losing clients lately, although not for any apparent invidious reasons. For most of these clients, he has recommended termination in view of their progress or his doubts about his ability to do for and with them more than he has. In Ms. Cabel's case, he doubts the wisdom of her action since she seems to be at a point of more durable problem resolution and increased capacity to cope with her problems if they recur.

Applicable Principles of Ethics

The principle of respect for the client's right to self-determination applies in this situation, as does the social worker's ethical responsibility to make her records promptly available to the replacing social worker, as she requests. Also applicable are the primacy of the client's interests and her right to know what is contained in her treatment records.

Priority of Applicable Principles

Ms. Cabel's self-determination merits high priority. Her best interests must also be considered, as must cooperation with Ms. Worth in Ms. Cabel's interest and at her request.

Risks to Be Taken into Account and Provided For

Premature or inappropriate transfer to Ms. Worth might, under some circumstances, represent a risk of progress reversal for Ms. Cabel. There is some risk for her in the transmission of the summary to Ms. Worth, if inappropriate reliance is placed on it. There is also risk of upsetting Ms. Cabel, in making her aware of its contents, if she is not already aware of them. She also risks Mr. Willet's negligence or delay in transmitting the requested summary, and whatever consequences that may have for her and for Ms. Worth's work with her.

As far as Mr. Willet is concerned, he stands to lose another client with risk for Ms. Cabel in what that may tempt him to do. If he is suffering financial difficulties, for example, or if his ego compels him to do what he can to keep her in treatment with him, ostensibly to attain complete success, he may compromise Ms. Cabel's self-determination.

Superseding Values

Under some circumstances — a replacement social worker who was adjudicated as unethical, for example — an appreciable hazard for Ms. Cabel might be regarded as sufficiently compelling to override Mr. Willet's normal responsibility to respect and act promptly upon Ms. Cabel's right to self-determination.

Provisions and Precautions

Mr. Willet might validly pose for Ms. Cabel such considerations that she might wish to take into account when making her final decision, but with great care lest she be moved more by his influence than by her own interests and priorities.

The summary that Mr. Willet prepares, if Ms. Cabel acts on her resolution to make the change, should be promptly forwarded to Ms. Worth. It should be limited to those essentials that Ms. Worth should be made aware of for suitable and timely initiation of an effective working relationship with Ms. Cabel. When preparing the summary, which Ms. Cabel should be free to read, Mr. Willet should carefully consider the potential impact of its contents and phrasing on Ms. Cabel. Optimally, it should contain nothing that would be entirely new to Ms. Cabel.

Evaluation

The process of transferring Ms. Cabel to Ms. Worth can be very emotionally charged. Great sensitivity and self-awareness are required on Mr. Willet's part so that what he says, and what he writes in the summary, do not, in their intonations and juxtapositions, convey thoughts or intentions inconsistent with Ms. Cabel's unhampered choice, and her prospects for a satisfactory working relationship with Ms. Worth.

DOING BUSINESS WITH
OR ON BEHALF OF CLIENTS

Ms. Carlson, a widow, suffers from a serious chronic illness and is in imminent danger of becoming mentally incompetent. Mistrusting her few remaining distant relatives, and having no close friends, Ms. Carlson appeals to Mr. Wald, the social worker in her nursing home with whom she has developed a close working relationship, to act on her behalf with power of attorney, and to take responsibility for the management of her financial assets and liabilities.

Applicable Principles of Ethics

Social workers should not enter into business transactions or relationships with clients that do not bear directly upon their professional treatment relationship. They have the ethical responsibility to avoid even the slightest hint or suggestion of improper use of influence on clients for purposes not directly related to professional objectives.

Priority of Applicable Principles

The focus of Mr. Wald's work and relationship with Ms. Carlson is on those needs that are appropriate subject matter of Mr. Wald's assigned social work responsibility and appropriate for Mr. Wald's skill and knowledge. The exercise of dominion over Ms. Carlson's financial affairs is precluded.

Risks to Be Taken into Account
and Provided For

For Mr. Wald to agree to Ms. Carlson's request is to risk confusion of Mr. Wald's assigned professional role and professional relationship with her. It also risks the appearance of improper use of Mr. Wald's influence on her, and perhaps the appearance of intent to profit from her trust in him. Agreeing to Ms. Carlson's request also introduces the risk of expectations and suspicions on Ms. Carlson's part that are inimical to the professional social work mission in which they are supposed to be engaged. As an employee of the nursing home, moreover, Mr. Wald risks the assumption of a function that is alien to that assigned to him and that is hazardous for the reputation and credibility of the nursing home.

Superseding Values

Although Ms. Carlson's peace of mind regarding her finances is valued, it does not supersede Mr. Wald's scrupulous adherence to the principles of social work ethics that apply in this situation.

Provisions and Precautions

Mr. Wald should avoid any transaction with or on behalf of Ms. Carlson that gives Mr. Wald influence or control over Ms. Carlson or her possessions, even if she invites or encourages it. A power of attorney contradicts the major social work premise of clients' retention of control over their own lives and destinies. If Ms. Carlson risks loss of mental capacity sufficient for her to handle her own affairs, and if she needs and seeks provision for it, as she seems to, then Mr. Wald, in his social work capacity, can guide her to the appropriate resource to make the necessary arrangements under the appropriate juridical controls. Mr. Wald can make clear that doing so is not an evasion of responsibility, or a discrediting of Ms. Carlson's need and reasonable and sensible request. Rather, doing so is an acknowledgement of limitations to Mr. Wald's competence and function, and of a need better met elsewhere in her best interests. In any case, he could continue to act as her social worker and thus assuage any doubts about his continuing interest in her needs and well-being.

Evaluation

Clarity is required for a disciplined and functional relationship between social workers and their clients. Social workers must resist the temptation to respond to clients' pleas to enter into reciprocal relationships or transactions that are not directly related to their therapeutic mission and that are likely to be antithetical to it. A power of attorney is but one illustration of such a conversion. Others might be a client's invitation to invest in an enterprise; a client's offer to become an employee as a form of barter for professional services; the social worker acting as a go-between for two of his clients to meet socially or to conduct business.

PROFESSIONAL RELATIONSHIP

A very attractive young woman in her late twenties, Ms. Carter was very distressed and distraught. Within two years she had invested herself and her emotions in two relationships with young men who abruptly broke off with her after many intimations of intent to marry her. Her self-esteem was at a very low ebb. She blamed herself for her fate and was very pessimistic about her future prospects. She brooded over growing older as she approached her thirtieth birthday, and she brooded over her loneliness. These feelings were affecting her demeanor and her work as an executive secretary.

She came to Mr. Weil for social work help out of sheer desperation. She dreaded admitting what she thought of as the uncomplimentary truth about herself and her situation. Mr. Weil developed a relationship with Ms. Carter that proved very salutary for her. She recouped her poise and confidence to a great extent. She felt rescued and better equipped to cope with her need for an enduring and satisfactory relationship. For this, she was very grateful. She began to find herself fantasizing about a romantic liaison with Mr. Weil, himself a rather attractive bachelor who was not a little attracted to her sexually. She soon began to let Mr. Weil know, in almost imperceptible yet unmistakable ways, that she would welcome an opportunity for a personal and romantic relationship with him.

Applicable Principles of Ethics

The relationship between social worker and client must remain professional and focused on professional objectives in the client's interest. It must not be confused or contaminated by actions of a personal and sexual nature on the part of the social worker. The social worker, moreover, must not exploit the relationship for his own gratification or for ends that conflict with the client's treatment goals.

Priority of Applicable Principles

First and foremost, Mr. Weil has the ethical responsibility to not exploit the vulnerabilities of Ms. Carter. Rather, through his professional relationship with her, he should help her cope with them successfully in the interest of her own well-being. Sexual activity and a romantic linkage with Ms. Carter compromises Mr. Weil's objectivity and the primacy of Ms. Carter's interests for which he is ethically responsible.

Risks to Be Taken into Account and Provided For

The temptation to respond in kind to Ms. Carter's overtures, as Mr. Weil may perceive them, must be resisted whether or not he is mistaken about them. Immediate damage to their professional relationship is inflicted either way. Implied is Ms. Carter's deprivation of the treatment she has needed, and in the professional manner in which she has needed it. She also incurs the risk of reversing the progress she has made. Also likely is Ms. Carter's loss of trust in Mr. Weil as a helping person with a focus on the problem for which she has sought help rather than on sexual gratification. This is an especially pertinent consideration in view of the history and experience that brought her to him in the first place. Even if she were in fact convinced, as Mr. Weil seems to suspect, that a liaison with him is what she wants or craves, it is neither why she is in treatment with him nor why he is supposed to be treating her.

Superseding Values

In this practice situation, no value supersedes the values to which Mr. Weil is assumed to be committed as an ethical social worker. A social worker does not harm a client, take advantage of a client's trust and gratitude, or do anything that confuses their professional relationship or makes it less effective.

Provisions and Precautions

The classical ethical dictum that a practitioner should not harm a patient or client suggests an important caution for Mr. Weil, even if the prospect of harm is only speculative. The prospect of harm may, in fact, be assumed in these circumstances. Ms. Carter could very well be experiencing a transference reaction, and Mr. Weil might very well be equipped to analyze and deal therapeutically with it. Whether or not he should proceed to do so, however, should be determined on the basis of whether it is appropriate for the function of his relationship with Ms. Carter and whether that function is what Ms. Carter has, with full awareness and understanding, bargained for. As a social worker, Mr. Weil would have to be able to justify such a turn in his approach to practice not only on the basis of his qualifications, but also on the basis of the definition of his function as a social worker.

However much Mr. Weil believes Ms. Carter to be inviting his sexual response, or if he is simply tempted to engage in sexual activity with her whatever her intention, discretion would dictate termination of their relationship. Referral to another practitioner may be indicated. This would require precaution on Mr. Weil's part to avoid causing Ms. Carter to feel rejected again. Extreme sensitivity and tact would be necessary, with emphasis on serving Ms. Carter's best interests and on the progress she has made, which may make referral appropriate and timely.

The assumption that Mr. Weil might be tempted to make, that his sexual response would be therapeutic for Ms. Carter, would be illusory at best. If Ms. Carter permitted it, for example, or even encouraged it, Mr. Weil would be a reciprocating participant and partner in a sex act. Hence, he would manifestly no longer be participating in his relationship with Ms. Carter on a level distinguishable from that of a personal relationship. He would not be maintaining the distance and objectivity, or the independence of professional judgment, that social work ethics require. Were Mr. Weil to participate in the sex act with complete detachment, his participation would bear all the hallmarks of manipulation and thus be inherently unethical. As suggested, if he is altogether mistaken about Ms. Carter's wishes or intentions, the professional cause is altogether lost. As a potential disruption and deprivation of service for Ms. Carter, and a likely loss of her trust not only in him but in social work in general, his reaction is unethical on several counts.

Under the circumstances, the most ethically commendable precaution is for Mr. Weil to remain convincingly above reproach and, if he can't, to find Ms. Carter a better venue for her purposes.

Evaluation

Mr. Weil's resistance to sexual temptation, whatever precipitates it, and his not exploiting Ms. Carter's possible vulnerabilities, are critical dimensions of his professional ethics. He is not supposed to take advantage of her need for treatment, and her vulnerability in seeking it. Nor is he supposed to behave in any fashion that impedes the initiation and maintenance of a relationship that ensures independence of professional judgment and the use of professional skill in Ms. Carter's best long-range interests. Sexual overtures or sexual activity would contaminate both. In this situation, such conduct, in addition to being unethical on its face, would be antithetical to the client's preeminent need as she presents it.

CONDITIONAL SERVICE

The Corloffs, a Russian Jewish family consisting of parents and two small children, obtained an exit visa from the Soviet Union. After waiting in Russia for six years under demeaning conditions, they were detained at a European transfer center for several months pending arrangements for immigration to the United States. After being denied immediate entry into the United States, which was what they preferred, they were cajoled by officials of an international Jewish agency into opting for immigration to Israel, with the promise of prompt action. Restrictions by United States authorities were finally lifted, however, and the Corloffs immigrated to the United States.

In the United States, the Corloffs were clients of the Arlow Immigration Service, sponsored and supported by the Jewish community. The goals of this agency included inducing and facilitating their identification as Jews. Ms. Weber, the social worker at the immigration service, was aware of the Corloffs' history and was charged with providing for their adjustment to their new environment until they could manage on their own. She was also responsible for arranging opportunities for their religious and cultural indoctrination and education, opportunities which the Corloffs continued to resist, having no inclination to engage in religious and cultural activities.

Applicable Principles of Ethics

Along with the primacy of clients' interests, principles of social work ethics that guide the social worker's practice include the right to self-determination and religious and cultural preferences. At the same time, the social worker is accountable for the competent performance of her assigned functions, and for the implementation of her employing agency's avowed goals.

Priority of Applicable Principles

As an employee of the Arlow Immigration Service, Ms. Weber is ethically responsible to aim for the achievement of its goals, and to perform her role in implementing the purposes for which the Jewish community has established and continues to support the agency. Included among these goals and purposes are those related to the Corloff family's religious and cultural orientation and education. As a service agency, however, the Arlow Immigration Service has also been charged with providing services and resources the Corloff family need for their adjustment and adaptation to their new environment. In view of the emphasis by the Jewish community on the liberation of families like the Corloffs from the oppression and constriction of the Soviet Union's totalitarian regime at the time — albeit with the hope that they would have the freedom and the interest to connect themselves to Jewish life and culture — Ms. Weber owes particular priority to their basic needs during their acclimation.

Risks to Be Taken into Account and Provided For

In a new land, the Corloff family are dependent upon Ms. Weber and the Arlow Immigration Service for their upkeep and help in their transition from a politically and religiously restrictive country to a relatively free and permissive one. As such, the Corloffs are prone to artificial passivity, and to submissiveness, lest they find themselves deprived of the services and resources they need. Their resistance to religious and cultural opportunities may impress Ms. Weber as ingratitude and arrogance when it may simply be a function of the years of living in a country with extreme antipathy to religion and democratic processes. As a result—all the more so if her own religious and cultural identification is especially pronounced—Ms. Weber may find herself responding critically if not punitively to the family's resistance and failure to capitalize on the opportunities Ms. Weber works hard to make available. Because of the Corloff family's experience since their departure from the Soviet Union, and implications of pressure on Ms. Weber's part, the Corloffs may begin to wonder whose purposes the Arlow Immigration Service program is really designed to serve.

Superseding Values

The Jewish community and the Arlow Immigration Service may regard the Jewish identification of the Corloff family as of primary concern. However, since the Corloffs are clients in need, and eligible to receive the basic services, the ethical responsibility of the Arlow Immigration Service, and therefore of Ms. Weber, to provide for them merits precedence. This carries the implication of concern about the Corloff family's dignity, preferences, and self-determination.

Provisions and Precautions

Ms. Weber does have the ethical responsibility to be guided in her practice by the agency goals and purposes for which she has assumed professional responsibility. These goals and purposes reflect the agency's and the Jewish community's interest in preserving, perpetuating, and perhaps enriching Jewish religion and culture. But they also relate to the welfare of the Corloff family. Aside from the agency rules and policies that affect eligibility for service, and that affect all clients without discrimination, the service offered to the Corloff family is not conditional upon their participation in religious and cultural practices. Their release from the Soviet Union and their immigration to the United States are identified as personal liberation, whatever the ultimate desire that motivates the Jewish community and Arlow Immigration Service.

Ms. Weber is professionally obliged to provide, and encourage the Corloff family's use of, resources and facilities that might help or even influence the Corloff family's connection to Jewish life and culture. However, she must do so with care to not judge them adversely, either actually or by intimation, or to in any way deprive them of their entitlements, or otherwise penalize them if they choose not to use them.

Evaluation

Agency services offered administratively to eligible clients are meant for those to whom they are offered and for whom they are designed, whatever the other incidental aspirations envisaged for them by others. Clients do not perforce become the vehicle for the realization of such incidental aspirations at the expense of their normal rights and prerogatives.

APPEARANCES

Shortly before the deadline for submission of bids on alterations and renovations at the Atlas Community Center, Mr. Prescott, the president of the City Construction Company, telephoned the Center's executive Mr. Winston, a social worker, to ask apologetically if he could drop his company's estimate off at Mr. Winston's home. He planned to be out of the city and wanted to be sure to get the estimate in on time for consideration by the Center's Board of Directors. Besides, he added, there were a few things that he would like an opportunity to mention to Mr. Winston. Both Mr. Prescott and Mr. Winston know that Mr. Winston carries a lot of weight with the Center's Board.

Applicable Principles of Ethics

As managing officer of an agency, the social work executive has the ethical responsibility to manage the agency in the most effective, efficient, and economical manner. This includes informed and objective appraisal of bids, estimates, and specifications — with expert help if necessary — for work to be done in the agency.

As a social worker with the agency's Board of Directors, the executive also has the ethical responsibility to ensure that the Board, in its policy-making and decision-making functions, has genuine autonomy in the context of its responsibility as agency and community trustee. In addition, the executive has the ethical responsibility to ensure provision for fairness, equity, and impartiality in the consideration and evaluation of bids and estimates, and to use his professional skill to do so.

Priority of Applicable Principles

Since Mr. Winston's defined professional function is to manage the Atlas Community Center effectively, efficiently, and economically, he owes priority to competent, informed, objective, and thorough implementation of the process of inviting and considering bids for work to be done. In the performance of his function with the Board, Mr. Winston also has the ethical responsibility to not impede the Board's opportunities to make decisions for which it is accountable and authorized. He is obligated to use his professional skill to assist Board members in the process. In dealing with contractors, Mr. Winston has the ethical responsibility to ensure fair and equitable treatment through the means at his official disposal, while safeguarding the Center's interests.

Risks to Be Taken into Account and Provided For

In the Board's exercise of its authorized discretion, the risk for the Atlas Community Center is that the Board's decisions and actions may not harmonize sufficiently with the Center's interests, policies, or public relations, or with the Center's obligation to give fair and equitable consideration to all bids.

If Mr. Winston agrees to receive Mr. Prescott's bid at his home after hours, and to discuss it with him without the knowledge and consent of the Board, Mr. Winston incurs the risk of appearing to favor City Construction Company, thus compromising his credibility and intruding on the Board's autonomy.

Superseding Values

Nothing in this situation, as presented, suggests any values that would justify neglect of Mr. Winston's ethical responsibility to the Atlas Community Center, its Board, or Mr. Prescott; nor would fulfilling that responsibility to any of them conflict with the responsibility to all of them.

Provisions and Precautions

To be ethical, Mr. Winston must avoid even the appearance of wrongdoing or of exceeding the boundaries of his assigned authority and responsibility. He must also avoid any implication of bias, favoritism, or undue influence, in the invitation and consideration of bids and subsequent action on them. More affirmatively, he must make clear to bidders and others the locus of authority for action on bids and the procedure for their consideration.

These constraints do not obviate Mr. Winston's opportunity to use his social work skills as well as courtesy and tact in guiding Mr. Prescott toward a more appropriate solution to his problem, if he has one, and to call it to the attention of available Board officers. In its consideration of bids, he provides the Board such guidance and resources as necessary for fair and sound decision-making consistent with the Center's procedures, policies, and interests, and with full knowledge that the Board may nevertheless err. However, since Mr. Winston is still accountable for the management of the Center, he plays his role on the Board with all the vigor and emphasis that might be required to prevent the Board from overlooking any detail that might make a difference in the choice it makes. He might do well to have such differences as he may have with the Board in the Board's records, recognizing that he, too, can err. For effective ethics, as for effective practice, productive working relationships between Mr. Winston and the Board are indispensable.

Evaluation

Whether or not Mr. Winston has actual authority to receive Mr. Prescott's bid, he retains responsibility for the management of the Atlas Community Center and for working with the Center's Board so that it can fulfill its responsibility in and to the Center. The important caution here is to be as concerned about the appearance of less than ethical conduct as about its actuality, and about the appearance of conduct inconsistent with assigned responsibility and authority. In this situation, social work ethics and social work practice coincide.

LOYALTY TO CLIENT VERSUS LOYALTY TO EMPLOYER

Mr. Carlysle, an employee of the Scott Company, is in treatment with Mr. Wayne, the social worker in the company's Employee Assistance Program. During one of their sessions, Mr. Carlysle reveals that he has tested positive for the AIDS virus. He does not wish to have this known in the company for fear of harassment by his peers and the possible loss of his job. In view of discussions by the company's management about testing employees for drugs and for the AIDS virus, Mr. Wayne suspects the loss of Mr. Carlysle's job to be a real possibility. However, the employees' union has geared itself for opposition to the testing plan during forthcoming labor-management negotiations.

Applicable Principles of Ethics

As an employee, the social worker in an Employee Assistance Program owes loyalty to his employer, and competent performance of his assigned function, which is to help employees (at their request) with problems that may be interfering with their work. As a social worker in a treatment relationship with clients, he also owes loyalty to clients. The principle of confidentiality applies to their relationship. Also applicable is the social worker's professional responsibility to prevent and oppose discrimination in the workplace.

Priority of Applicable Principles

Although Mr. Wayne is accountable to the Scott Company for the competent performance of his assigned function, his practice as a social worker commits him to the principles of social work ethics associated with it. Among these, the principle of confidentiality merits highest priority.

Risks to Be Taken into Account and Provided For

Mr. Carlysle risks exposure of his secret, with potentially troubling consequences, by virtue of his resort to the Scott Company's Employee Assistance Program for service. The risk also exists that Mr. Carlysle's condition will be discovered if the Scott Company's management succeeds in introducing a testing program. This would also deprive him and other company personnel of their privacy and perhaps their jobs, depending on the effectiveness of the legal protections available to them.

Superseding Values

No value relevant to this situation supersedes the values to which Mr. Wayne is ethically committed in his relationship to Mr. Carlysle.

Provisions and Precautions

Mr. Carlysle's revelation, in confidence, to Mr. Wayne has no bearing on his job in Scott Company or on its administrative policies. Mr. Wayne's practice with him is theretofore consistent with his professional function in the company's Employee Assistance Program.

Mr. Wayne should provide the help and guidance Mr. Carlysle may need to deal with any consequences his situation may have for him. He should neither reveal, nor urge Mr. Carlysle to reveal, the fact that he is HIV positive. He should make it clear that he regards that to be Mr. Carlysle's choice, and apprise him of the considerations and consequences to take into account. Mr. Wayne should also prepare himself and Mr. Carlysle for the action that may be necessary to forestall the introduction of a testing program by the

Scott Company, and for what Mr. Carlysle and others may experience or need to do if the program is introduced.

Mr. Wayne does account for the time spent in treating Mr. Carlysle, as the Scott Company requires, but without specifying details about the substance of the treatment or resulting revelations, a practice that would be indicated for all his cases.

Evaluation

The Scott Company's proffer of Mr. Wayne's services through the Employee Assistance Program is designed to make the needed social work treatment available to Mr. Carlysle and other employees. In making it available, the Scott Company does count on it to ultimately serve the company's purposes as well, since healthy, well-adjusted, and untroubled employees are more effective employees. However, Mr. Carlysle does not relinquish his right to privacy by seeking it. As a social worker, Mr. Wayne respects that right, and respects the confidences that Mr. Carlysle entrusts to him.

Employee Assistance Programs are intended for employees who use them. Social workers who are treating employees owe their employers an accounting of the fact that they are doing so, but not what they are treating them for, or other confidential details of the treatment process. Employees need the demonstrated assurance that they will not be penalized for using the service. Social workers, in turn, need the demonstrated assurance that they can perform their assigned function ethically. Any limiting conditions that are set for either social worker or clients in the service must be clearly stated so that each can choose whether or not to participate.

SOCIAL WORK STUDENTS AND STRIKES

Ms. Soren is a social work field instructor employed by the Silcott School of Social Work to supervise a unit of social work students in the Astor Social Agency. After attempting to negotiate a new contract without success, the staff of the agency goes out on strike and pickets the agency. Some of the students identify with the strikers and intend to honor the picket line. Others are opposed to doing so, and still others are uncertain about their prerogatives since

they are students placed in the agency for the purposes of professional social work education.

Applicable Principles of Ethics

The social work school and the field instructor have the ethical
responsibility to ensure for students, placed in an agency for supervised field practice, learning opportunities conducive to acquisition
of the knowledge, skills, and attitudes required for competent and
ethical social work practice. Moreover, the field instructor as a
member of the school's faculty, has the ethical responsibility to not
use the entree permitted her by the agency to subvert the purposes
of either the agency or the striking staff.

Priority of Applicable Principles

The predominant responsibility of both the Silcott School of Social Work and Ms. Soren is to provide for the professional education of social work students. Ms. Soren also has the ethical responsibility to provide the oversight and controls necessary for the
protection of the Astor Social Agency's clients who are assigned to
the students, and for the assurance of competent service to them. In
addition, Ms. Soren has the ethical responsibility to monitor students' use of the agency's resources and their adherence to agency
policies. Moreover, Ms. Soren has the ethical responsibility to prevent alignments by students with either the Astor Social Agency or
the striking staff, that are inappropriate for their status as students
invited by the agency to study social work.

Risks to Be Taken into Account
and Provided For

Whatever their predisposition in relation to the strike and the
picket line — whether to cross the picket line or to honor it, for example — students risk becoming caught up in labor-management
strife to which they are not party. They are also liable to find themselves in educationally unproductive conflicts both among themselves and between themselves and Ms. Soren and others, because
of opposing views only extraneously related to the educational purposes for which they are in the Astor Social Agency. They also risk
alienation from the Astor Social Agency or the staff, and residual

animosity that might interfere with the use of the agency as a field instruction placement after the strike has been settled, however satisfactorily. On the other hand, the combative atmosphere of the Astor Social Agency during the strike is likely to adversely affect the educational opportunities of students.

Superseding Values

Since the primary purpose of both the placement of students in the Astor Social Agency for field instruction and the assignment to Ms. Soren of supervisory responsibility for them is their professional education, that remains the major consideration for all the parties involved and affected. Other values, like equitable resolution of the strike, require consideration, but not to the extent of obviating or diluting Ms. Soren's primary ethical responsibilities.

Provisions and Precautions

A major objective for the Silcott School of Social Work and Ms. Soren would be to avoid subjecting the students to conflicts of choice regarding the strike, or the agonies of ambivalence and uncertainty about it. Their status as students plausibly exempts them from responsibility in relation to the strike. Withdrawing them from the Astor Social Agency, with a declaration of neutrality and the expressed wish for the speedy resolution of the strike for the sake of service to clients and the education of students, would carry the least emotional charge with the fewest adverse consequences for the relationship between the Silcott School of Social Work and the Astor Social Agency. In addition, students are thus sheltered from a potentially destructive and educationally dysfunctional professional experience.

Constructive use can be made of the resulting gap in the students' agency experience by educational consideration of strikes and labor-management relations in social agencies; the nature, utilization, and functions of conflict; and the place of unions in professions like social work. Other alternative educational opportunities could also be afforded to students at the school and in other settings. Plans and arrangements could also be made for students' resumption of supervised practice-oriented responsibilities in other settings should the strike last long enough to deny them optimal opportunities to achieve the educational goals envisaged for them. Incumbent on the Astor Social Agency would be the responsibility—perhaps with the cooperation of the striking staff—to provide for emergencies affecting clients.

Evaluation

The actions contemplated are consistent with the more compelling ethical responsibilities of school, students, and field instructor in relation to the Astor Social Agency and its clients. All share responsibility for providing opportunities and conditions conducive to preparing students for competent and ethical social work practice. Moreover, the actions contemplated would not intrude unduly on the options, rights, and responsibilities of the parties to the labor-management conflict.

CLASSROOM REVELATIONS

Ms. Winthrop conducts a social work practice course at the Strean Graduate School of Social Work. Ms. Wendell is a student in her final year of the master's degree program in social work. She prepares a record of her practice at the Acton Agency—where she has been placed for field instruction—for classroom discussion. In this record she reveals agency practices of an unethical nature, and practices detrimental to the agency's clientele. The work of her field instructor, Mr. Solar, also leaves much to be desired in that he frequently misses supervisory conferences with Ms. Wendell. Those in which he does participate reflect considerable incompetence and negligence. At the same time, Ms. Wendell reveals extensive inadequacies of her own, including insufficient awareness of the limitations and problems implicit in the content of her recording.

Applicable Principles of Ethics

The principles of confidentiality and academic freedom apply to classroom discussion of agency practices and experience. Revelations about a field instruction agency made by a social work student (who is given access to information about it for the purposes of social work education) are not properly (ethically) used against the agency by either the student or the social work school which places the student in the agency. The student's revelations, made for the purposes of classroom discussion, are also not properly used against the student.

On the other hand, social workers have the ethical responsibility to discourage and prevent agency personnel practices that are detrimental or harmful to the agency's clientele. Social work schools, moreover, have the ethical responsibility to avoid field instruction placements that may limit students' learning opportunities, or even be antithetical to their acquisition of knowledge and their development of skills for competent and ethical social work practice.

As a social worker and member of the social work profession, as well as a teacher in a professional school, the classroom instructor also has the ethical responsibility to make well-considered educational judgments regarding the academic performance of students and their suitability as candidates for careers in social work.

Priority of Applicable Principles

The principle of confidentiality, as it applies to the Acton Agency and to Ms. Wendell, is virtually sacrosanct. Considerations that contravene this principle must be very compelling. Nevertheless, ethical responsibility to clients, and to Ms. Wendell in relation to the quality and conditions of her professional education, is also shared by the Strean School, Ms. Winthrop, the Acton Agency, and Mr. Solar.

Risks to Be Taken into Account and Provided For

The Acton Agency, Mr. Solar, and Ms. Wendell risk victimizing themselves by exposing themselves to observation, critical appraisal, possible serious penalties through actions taken and revelations volunteered for the purpose of social work education. Through faulty agency practices, poor educational experiences, and inadequate monitoring and evaluation of Ms. Wendell's work, there are risks for both the agency's clients and future clients of Ms. Wendell.

Superseding Values

Trust in Ms. Winthrop, the classroom instructor, and a classroom atmosphere of academic freedom and candor, are highly valued in our society. Therefore the resulting danger of self-incrimination may be important enough to warrant tempering application of the principles of ethics attributed to the various participants in this situation.

Provisions and Precautions

Victimizing the participants (in the various ways to which they are subject) because of revelations volunteered or made possible in the service of Ms. Wendell's professional education needs to be avoided. Ms. Winthrop should use the revelations in Ms. Wendell's recording (and the classroom discussion that flows from it) only for the achievement of classroom purposes. Ms. Wendell's classmates should also be apprised of their responsibility to keep the substance of both confidential.

Ms. Winthrop's evaluation of Ms. Wendell should be based, not on the content of her recording or the quality of her work in the agency which it reflects, but on the manner and conduct of her presentation and discussion in the classroom. Ms. Wendell's performance in the fulfillment of other class requirements should also be considered.

In view of the superseding value considerations, alternative sources of more directly available information about the Acton Agency, field instructor Mr. Solar, and Ms. Wendell must be used in order for Ms. Winthrop and the Strean School of Social Work to act upon their ethical responsibility to the Acton Agency's clients and others adversely affected (both in actuality and in prospect). One of the issues the Strean School of Social Work would have to contend with, on the basis of all the information at its disposal without relying on classroom revelations, is whether to transfer Ms. Wendell from the Acton Agency to another placement. There she might gain a more satisfactory learning experience, and be evaluated on the basis of a more accurate measure of her ability and performance if there is uncertainty about them. The Strean School of Social Work must also decide whether to use the Acton Agency as a field placement in the future. Such decisions would require a well-founded process of exchange and communication, and participation by all the affected parties.

Evaluation

Because the Acton Agency's, and the field instructor, Mr. Solar's practices persist as matters of ethical concern, they require further attention. However, means other than the direct and immediate use of Ms. Wendell's classroom revelations are necessary. This may make timely action difficult as a result, but to invite candor for the purposes of classroom discussion only to penalize it is a form of entrapment. The education of Ms. Wendell remains a prime concern, as do fair testing and an accurate appraisal of her ability and performance, both for her sake, and for the sake of those she may be destined to serve.

DECEPTIVE RESEARCH

Mr. Werner, a social worker and a professor eager for tenure and promotion, was concerned about his university's pressure on faculty to conduct research and accrue publications. He designed an inquiry to determine whether editors of scholarly social work journals were influenced by the results of reported social work research in evaluating manuscripts submitted for publication. His plan was to invent a research report in two versions, one showing positive results of a social work practice method; the other, negative or neutral results. His purpose was to demonstrate an editorial bias toward the publication of manuscripts reporting positive results.

Applicable Principles of Ethics

Social workers have the ethical responsibility to conduct or collaborate in research, and to be aware of and apply research relevant to their social work practice. They are also expected to participate or cooperate in the advancement of social work knowledge. Social workers who conduct and report research are ethically committed to the conventions of scholarly research. In addition to using acceptable procedures associated with credible and creditable research, they are expected to avoid destructive and deceptive inquiries, especially those harmful to subjects and participants, and those in which subjects and participants have been maneuvered into participation without their informed consent.

Priority of Applicable Principles

In his conduct of research, the primary ethical responsibility of Mr. Werner is to avoid harming or misleading subjects and those who use and rely on his research. He is also ethically responsible to adhere to research procedures that are designed for authenticity of results, and to indicate limitations that characterize their application and affect the results. Honesty, accuracy, and objectivity in reporting his research are additional principles to which he is assumed to be committed.

Risks to Be Taken into Account and Provided For

The pressure on Mr. Werner to conduct research is apt to color his judgment when choosing and executing a research project. The fabrication of research results in two versions risks publication and diffusion of either or both. It also risks the reliance of others on the research, with potentially damaging consequences for researchers and consumers of research. There is a further risk of misleading editors who, in good faith, treat the reports as legitimate and accurate, causing embarrassment and error for them.

Superseding Values

No particular value is suggested that warrants the violation of principles of ethics for which Mr. Werner is accountable. On the other hand, neither does his responsibility for the advancement of social work knowledge and practice nor for testing them take precedence over his responsibility for truth in his conduct of research.

Provisions and Precautions

Responding to pressure for the purpose of professional advancement is a red flag to caution Mr. Werner against ill-conceived or insufficiently considered research, and shortcuts or deceptions in its conduct. Resorting to deceptive reports in order to test for editorial bias (however interesting and illuminating that might appear to be) is an insufficient and unethical reason for pursuing an inquiry that may have damaging consequences for consumers and others who rely on it. If Mr. Werner's research question is compelling enough for Mr. Werner and the social work profession, other, more ethically acceptable, means would be preferable.

Evaluation

Mr. Werner might feel unduly hampered by the constraints and constrictions to which he is ethically subject. However, the kind of research procedure he has in mind is not justifiable, whatever the value of his project. The major problem is not the embarrassment he might cause for editors, although, as a matter of responsibility to colleagues, it cannot be cavalierly dismissed. The chief concerns are those for truth and accuracy in research reports submitted for publication, and about readers' reliance on them.

WHISTLE-BLOWING

Mr. Wallach is a social work supervisor in the Division of Services to Children of the Municipal Welfare Department. He is concerned about confirmed incidents of staff negligence and incompetence which have afflicted services to children. The result has been injury and death for many children who have been repeatedly and violently abused by parents and other caretakers. He has resorted to all the administrative channels available to him to effect change in the situation, but without success.

Applicable Principles of Ethics

Social workers have an ethical as well as administrative responsibility to adhere to the policies and procedures of the social agencies by which they are employed. They are also expected to respect the confidences of these agencies and their staffs, and of their clienteles. The principle of client self-determination also applies as it affects the preferences of agency clients.

Priority of Applicable Principles

As an employee of the Division of Services to Children, and as a condition of his employment, Mr. Wallach is expected to work within the framework of the Division's policies and procedures. As a social worker and as an employee, Mr. Wallach is also ethically responsible to preserve the confidences of Division colleagues and clients.

Risks to Be Taken into Account and Provided For

Mr. Wallach's neglect of his responsibilities to the Division and to colleagues can undermine their work and their services. Failure to respect the confidences of clients, whether conveyed directly to Mr. Wallach or to others in the Division, would undermine their trust in the Division and damage their relationships to its personnel. The children the Division serves, however, are also at great risk not only from injury if the abuse they may be experiencing is neglected, but also possibly more serious harm from intimidating parents or caretakers if the fact of the abuse is revealed to the authorities.

Superseding Values

The welfare and lives of apparently defenseless children are at stake in this situation. The valuation of their well-being is a preeminent value for Mr. Wallach as a social worker. Therefore, the violation of principles of ethics for which he is directly accountable in relation to the Division and his colleagues would appear to be justified, whether the clients he is concerned about are under his direct care or not.

Provisions and Precautions

Having verified the existence of abuse, staff neglect and incompetence and having exhausted all his opportunities and all the avenues of change available to him in the Division of Services to Children, Mr. Wallach would be justified in resorting to the hierarchy in the Municipal Welfare Department for action on the problems. Failing in that attempt, he would then be justified in resorting to the locality's administration for intervention. If that, too, fails, then Mr. Wallach would be justified in going outside to any resource (including the media, if necessary) that might have a helpful effect. He should keep in mind the caution, in each case, that specific identities of clients not be revealed and that only such information be shared as would at least precipitate prompt inquiry and investigation, and protection for endangered children.

These actions would have to be regarded as violations of Mr. Wallach's ethical responsibility to the Division and to his colleagues, but violations in response to the priority assigned to the welfare of the children at risk. For Mr. Wallach, this would add the risk of censure and possible loss of his job. He would be advised, therefore, to anticipate and provide for personal consequences. But, the prospect of such penalties for blowing the whistle is a reminder that one must be very clear about one's facts as well as convictions in such a situation, in order to have the confidence and courage to act on them. (The law may also have something to say about what is expected.)

Evaluation

The choices for Mr. Wallach are extremely difficult, and the proposed actions could be very unpleasant and painful, but measures to protect defenseless and endangered children require all the courage and perseverance that can be mustered. The ideology of the social work profession — the values to which social workers are presumed to aspire — inspires as much.

Chapter V

Learning and Teaching Ethics
for Social Work Practice and Education

SUPERVISORS AND TEACHERS
AS MENTORS AND MODELS

Social workers who orient, indoctrinate, train, supervise, teach, and consult with volunteers, staff members, students, and others who practice social work (or aspire to do so), or who manage social services, have both the responsibility and opportunity to teach, inspire, and represent social work ethics.

Whatever the role or status of those whom social workers are in a position to affect or influence—that is, those who are program or administrative volunteers; paraprofessionals, professionals; undergraduate, graduate, or advanced students; or teachers—for them, the social workers are both mentors and models. They have the responsibility, and they have the opportunity, to communicate to them the substance and import of ethics, and the relevance of ethics to their roles and to social work practice and functions in general. They also have the responsibility, and the opportunity, to represent and demonstrate, in the process, their own ethics as they apply to the performance of their own roles.

At the very least, by their words, references, and illustrations—as well as by their own example—social workers begin to raise the consciousness of those they work with, regarding the functions and the necessity of ethics in social work and social work-related endeavors and activities, including their own.

Whatever the substance and the goals of the activities in which individuals are engaged as volunteers, trainees, staff members, or students, emphasis on the values implicated in the activities affords opportunities for them to contemplate and contend with their duties and obligations in them.

A major objective of orienting, training, supervising, and teaching others to perform social work and social-work related roles and functions is to awaken their sensibilities regarding the moral implications of those roles and functions. The policies and decisions they are empowered to make as agency board members, for example, may be examined from the point of view of the dignity of the persons affected as well as responsiveness to budgetary realities and constraints.

On the other hand, persons who provide services or who, in other ways, affect the fates and circumstances of others (clients and supervisees, for example) can be helped to attune themselves to the probable impact of their behavior. They can be shown how their behavior may be perceived by individuals who are in need, in crisis, or in jeopardy, and the ethical responsibility that implies.

In each case, there is knowledge to be acquired — about human need, human behavior, human conditions, human foibles, human frailties, and human vulnerabilities — and principles of ethics with which to become familiar (like confidentiality, self-determination, and prohibitions against abuse of power and exploitation). The expected level of knowledge and of skill mastery, when applying it in practice, will depend on the status and career aspirations of the learner, and the institutional context of the learning experience. The requirements, and the criteria for appraising and acting upon the achievements of agency board members, are of course different from those affecting social work students and staff members. So are the consequences. But each merits the effort and the attempt if social work ethics are to be served and diffused.

The higher the level of professional discretion that may be anticipated to be employed by a learner, either immediately or in the future (in private and independent practice, for example), the greater the mastery of knowledge and skill to be aimed for and to be required.

RELATING LEVEL OF ETHICAL MASTERY
TO LEVEL OF EDUCATION
AND RESPONSIBILITY

Volunteers

Program and service volunteers who deal with and affect clients and others directly (by providing services to them, for example) require awareness of principles of ethics since their performance of assigned tasks must be disciplined enough to avoid offenses to the rights, prerogatives, and vulnerabilities of others. They also require oversight by social workers charged with their supervision.

The objective of orienting administrative volunteers to the relevance of social work ethics to social services is primarily to acquaint them with the values to which social workers and social agencies are committed in relation to clients and others. The purpose is to sensitize administrative volunteers, like board members, to the ethical implications of their decisions and policies.

Apprentices and Paraprofessionals

For apprentices and paraprofessionals, instruction and supervision are required regarding the ethical aspects of their service roles and administrative relationships however limited. The boundaries to the initiative they are expected to exercise require delineation so that they understand how far they may or may not go in contending with issues of ethics that may emerge in their experience. They must also know how rapidly they are expected to resort to the help and intervention of those to whom they are administratively accountable. Educational opportunities, aside from available supervisory procedures, are essential in order to increase their awareness of the values that are integral components of the culture of their employing agencies and institutions, whatever the connection of those values to their own limited functions. In addition to such application as those values may have to their own assignments, they serve as indications of what would be in store were the apprentices and paraprofessionals to undertake more extensive professional careers as social workers. They may even be helped to decide whether such careers are for them at all, and whether they can identify with the kind of ideology implied.

Undergraduate Social Work Students

For students enrolled in Baccalaureate and Associate Degree social work programs, and particularly those for whom supervised field practice is prescribed as a part of their curriculum, a degree of mastery of social work ethics in practice as well as theory, although limited, is required and hence an important educational objective. In supervisory conferences and classroom instruction, students should be introduced to the rationale and to the fundamental principles of social work ethics, the need for which may be encountered by students in their actual experience. They will need such an orientation as a foundation of social work knowledge and skill. Here, too, administrative and educational controls will be necessary so that students will not be entirely on their own when confronting or anticipating complex practice situations. Allowances must always be made for differences in student capacity and readiness.

Graduate Social Work Students

Students enrolled in Master of Social Work degree programs within graduate schools and departments of social work are presumed to be committed to professional social work careers. The general educational objective is to help them become equipped for social work responsibility of a rather high order, if not immediately upon graduation then shortly after entry and induction into the profession. They need an opportunity for a realistic and systematic transition to professional employment and practice, preferably under competent and experienced guidance.

For some graduates — assuming adequate and promising achievement of degree requirements — responsibility for the supervision of other practitioners and personnel is likely, especially for those skilled in working with groups. For all graduates, whether or not they face the immediate prospect of supervisory or administrative responsibility of any substantial kind, educational objectives should include mastery of knowledge and development of skill for competent and ethical social work practice, with capacity for independent judgment to the extent that they may have to exercise it, if not immediately then somewhere along their vocational way. For those who are destined to supervise and teach others, an additional aspiration would be to help equip them, at least to some extent, for the important task of influencing the ethics as well as the competence of others.

Advanced Students

For students in advanced and doctoral social work education programs, the aim would be to provide opportunities to develop—and perhaps to develop further, since they may already be teachers, and are likely to be seasoned practitioners—their capacity to teach, and to inquire into, the substance and theory of social work ethics. Depending on inclination, aptitude, and career aspirations, students could be helped and encouraged to undertake study of approaches to curriculum planning and pedagogy for, and empirical and theoretical research into, professional ethics in general and social work ethics in particular. The focus, on one hand, could be on the conceptualization, derivation, and application of principles of professional and social work ethics; and, on the other hand, on modes of scholarly and philosophical inquiry into the sources, origins, and development of professional and social work ethics.

DEVELOPING SKILL FOR ETHICAL SOCIAL WORK PRACTICE AND EDUCATION: SUMMING UP

Whether through the use of the proposed paradigm or through other pedagogical means, social work students and staffs may be given opportunities to become aware of, and sensitive to, issues of ethics that may emerge at any juncture in social work practice. With effective guidance and stimulation, they may also become increasingly familiar with principles of social work ethics, and develop skill in their application.

At a minimum, the consciousness of students and staff regarding these issues and principles would be raised in classes, supervisory conferences, and in-service training sessions. As their own practice or experience is explored and discussed, the ethical implications of practice situations may be increasingly detected to alert students and staff to the operation of ethics in, and relevance of ethics to, the use of social work skills and knowledge. This includes the possibility that ethical imperatives may conflict with, and perhaps supersede, strictly-speaking practice and service goals. What may be regarded as ethically "right" may be accorded precedence over what may be regarded as practically better or more effective.

Discussion of practice experiences can help students and staff develop skill in the analysis of practice situations for improved discrimination between issues of practice (those affecting the attainment of service ends) and issues of ethics (those affecting conduct valued in practice without exclusive regard to what works best in practice). Assignments, institutes, symposia, and workshop exercises may be used, along with other work-related exchanges and interactions, to permit students and staff to hone their observational and practice skills in relation to both practice goals and ethics.

Content of classes, supervisory conferences, and in-service training sessions, as well as preparation for them, should include codes of social work ethics and other scholarly and practical resources to increase familiarity with the types of principles of ethics that exist and the complexities of their application. Opportunities for testing their ramifications and application should also be provided to students and staff. Provision should be made for an appreciation of the modulations and modifications of ethical principles that differences in responsibilities, clienteles, and circumstances may require. Students and staff can also be encouraged to participate in efforts and processes to amend and improve the content and implementation of existing codes of social work ethics, and thus to play their part in the larger social work scene.

First and foremost, perhaps, is the representation of values and ethics by instructors, supervisors, and administrators in all of their contacts and experiences with students and staff. Their own conduct can serve as model, example, and inspiration, as well as case material for inquisitive students and staff. Ultimately, of course, the performance of students and staff in their assigned professional roles should be noted and evaluated — by themselves if not by others—from the point of view of their ethics in addition to their professional skill and knowledge.

Many opportunities are available for self-generated acquisition and development of knowledge and skill for ethical practice and education. Through peer group supervision as well as peer group educational and consultation sessions, social workers in private practice can arrange their own opportunities. All it takes is a modicum of ingenuity, imagination, humility, and concern. Social work ethics are worth every bit and every kind of effort that can be put into them. A lot of people in and outside of the social work profession depend on them.

Index

T - #0591 - 101024 - C0 - 212/152/8 - PB - 9781560242833 - Gloss Lamination